Endorsements & Testimonials
for
Weight Solutions: The New Body-Mind-Spirit Approach

"The most complete book on healthy weight loss has finally arrived—a book that doesn't concentrate on the "bad" carbohydrates or the "good" proteins, but rather encourages one to take a holistic look at one's life experience. To include the mind, body, emotions, and spirit in an endeavor to lose weight is an equation for success. This sensible approach will not only insure weight loss, but will also increase the quality of one's life. *Weight Solutions* is a book that gently encourages the individual to be an active participant in their own healing. It is a book that I will be recommending to my patients who struggle with weight loss and yearn for a happier more gratifying life."
Dr. Jeffrey Kucine, DO
Osteopathic Physician

"A real how-to for healthy weight loss. A simple guide for truly healthful living. This work clearly expresses the knowledge of experienced clinicians."
Dr. Frederick Sutter, MD
Health Promotion and Musculoskeletal Specialist

"I have now been following your program for about seven weeks and have lost 20 pounds! Woo hoo! Your book is so easy to follow and I have become dependant on the shopping lists. Not only have I lost weight, I feel so much better now! Thank you for creating an easy to follow plan."
K.J.G.
Teacher

"[The book] spoke to me about health in ways I had not heard before. It provided the clarity of information to begin and the no-nonsense encouragement to get and stay in the driver's seat. I especially appreciate how you navigate the reader through the process of harmonizing body, mind and spirit. It is making a difference in my life."
A.M.M.
Business Professional

"I can see that simply following a diet doesn't work because of all the emotional energy around food. The mind-body-spirit approach you use is awesome. Eating right is a major lifestyle change and apparently takes A LOT of energy and support. Your book is wonderfully informative and simple and gives excellent resources for those who want to know more."
C.S.
Mother and Business Owner

Weight Solutions
The New
Body-Mind-Spirit Approach

A Workbook that Works!

By Janet Cunningham, Ph.D. and Judith Valentine, Ph.D.

Printed in the USA by Heritage Authors®
Published by Two Suns Press

Cover design by Janet Cunningham

Authors' Note: The information in this book reflects the authors' experience and is not intended to replace medial advice. It is not the intent of the authors to diagnose or prescribe. The intent is only to offer information to help you cooperate with your physician in your mutual quest for desirable health. Only your physician can determine whether or not this program is appropriate for you. Before embarking on this or any other program, you should consult your physician.

ISBN: 978-0-9640026-4-7

Other Books by Janet Cunningham:

Inner Selves: the Feminine* Path to Weight Loss (*for men and women who value their intuitive nature)
A Tribe Returned
Caution: Soul Mate Ahead! Co-authored with Michael Ranucci
Survival on a Wing and a Prayer, coauthored with Gail Lionetti
The Love's Fire Trilogy:
> *Book One: Love's Fire: Beyond Boundaries.* Co-authored with Tianna Conte-Dubs, N.D. and William
> *Book Two: Love's Fire: Living the Eternal Journey.* Co-authored with Tianna Conte-Dubs, N.D. and William
> *Book Three: Love's Fire: Initiation into the 21st Century.* Co-authored with Tianna Conte-Dubs, N.D. and William

Audio Programs:
Weight Loss Breakthroughs — a four audio-cassette workshop or two CDs

By Judith Valentine:

A Nutritional Guide to a Natural Menopause (publication in process)

Articles:

"Soft Drinks: America's *Other* Drinking Problem". *Wise Traditions,* Summer 2001.
"The Trouble with Low Fat Diets". *Annapolis Holistic Health Newsletter,* Spring 2000.
"A Continuing Series on Natural Menopause". *Annapolis Holistic Health Newsletter,* 1997–1999.

Table Of Contents

Dedication

We dedicate this book to you the reader, as you begin your journey through the miraculous freedom in weight management and improved health that this Plan offers.

Acknowledgments

We wish to acknowledge the several thousand clients and dieters who over the years have come to us in our individual practices and seminars. It is through you that we have expanded our knowledge, taking information beyond theory to practical application.

We especially wish to acknowledge Cheryl Hoxsie, who pushed us to move forward to get this information into print. Her questions and suggestions were enormously helpful.

In preparing our workbook, several colleagues and friends served as readers to provide feedback; a sincere thank you to each person: Dana Collins, Terri Diener and Susan Owen. We also both called upon our own sisters who contributed as readers and editors: Judith's sister, Linda Ellsworth, and Janet's sister, Judith Ann Burns.

Our information is based on more than 50 years of combined experience in our respective practices. In addition, it draws from the knowledge of others who are well known in the field of nutrition and weight loss, including Dr. Robert Atkins, Barry Sears and other low carbohydrate gurus; Lois Lindauer and The Diet Workshop program; Ideal Health and the MetPrep eating program; the dietary guidelines of Metagenics; and many others who are referenced in our program and in the Appendices.

We wish to express our deep appreciation to Felicia Barlow, the official editor of our book. Felicia's attention to detail, as well as questioning for clarification, became invaluable to the quality of the final publication.

Janet would like to acknowledge the talent of Nancy George-Grahlmann, illustrator of her book, *Inner Selves: The Feminine* Path to Weight Loss (*for men and women who value their intuitive nature)*. Six of Nancy's illustrations have been used in our workbook.

Judith would like to offer her gratitude to colleagues and clients who, during the last eight years, have held the clear vision of this book. A special appreciation goes to her husband, Barry Valentine, who insists he avoided an inevitable sinus surgery because of healthy changes he made to his overall nutrition and diet. We hope all of you have as much faith in your ability to ward off the inevitable.

Preface

Δ

Sometimes people meet and there is a spontaneous camaraderie. That was true for us. We have gone to each other as colleagues, seeking guidance, with respect for each other's expertise. As friends, we have supported and encouraged one another in personal and professional ventures. Joining in this endeavor to create a workbook for weight solutions seemed a natural step.

Many people have suffered for years due to misguided information related to dieting, or weight loss and nutrition. In fact, serious health risks, and even death, have resulted in the desperate search for an answer to obesity. Yes, the desire for a magic cure still exists. However, the past 40-plus years of weight-loss mania have proven that the sought-after overnight miracle is a myth. Today, people are not quite as eager to put complete faith in a diet doctor, weight-loss guru, or magazine advertisement.

On the other hand, currently there is more valid information available to the public related to eating and exercise. New food products that emphasize low fat, or low sugar have become a multimillion dollar industry. Gyms have sprung up in every town with an emphasis on machines that build the body. A new career category called "fitness trainers" has become a part of society and busy people consult with them in gyms or in the privacy of their home.

In the past several years, models, as well as entertainers, have gone from an average size 10 to size 4 or lower. Airbrushing in magazine photographs and movies is standard procedure. Yet, in spite of this enormous emphasis on the body, the average American of all ages is becoming fatter and fatter. Obesity is now acknowledged to be a national epidemic. Shocking statistics recently report that 60% of Americans are overweight. Less common, yet just as unhealthy, are those who are severely underweight.

In addition to food and exercise marketing, there is another point of confusion. This involves a flood of advertising and information related to nutritional supplements, herbs, and vitamins. Sounding somewhat like a snake-oil salesman, the salesperson claims everything from weight loss to energy to super-health and sexual vitality. The consumer is lost in a maze of guesswork in reading labels in health food stores, or non-discriminately taking vitamins because it seems like a good idea. One of the purposes for our workbook is to give you some basic and useful information related to nutrition. This is the expertise of Judith Valentine.

Perhaps the greatest breakthrough in the field of health has been scientific acceptance of what we have intuitively always known — the body and mind are intricately connected. Translating this knowledge into practical application, however, has been slow in coming.

Therefore, the second purpose of our workbook is to bring greater understanding about how your mind and emotions may be creating and holding onto body fat. This is the expertise of Janet Cunningham.

You will benefit most from this endeavor by creating a Workbook Support Group. This helps to sustain motivation and achieve realistic goals. A synergy of creative forces is unleashed in joining together with similar intentions.

The New Body-Mind-Spirit Approach for Weight Solutions was born by our joining together. We wish to bring to your awareness the fact that your body is the vehicle for your soul. Whatever your spiritual beliefs may be, care for your body — this vehicle, or temple — is important to your soul's journey. The care of your mind is also important to your physical and spiritual well being.

We trust that in this workbook you will find solutions to your overweight or underweight issues. We sincerely hope that these new discoveries will bring more health, peace and joy to your body, mind and spirit. We believe in you!

Janet Cunningham, Ph.D. and Judith Valentine, Ph.D.

Introduction
To the New Body-Mind-Spirit
Approach
Δ

Your Body

Knowledge of nutrition science and its relationship to our health is a constantly evolving process. As we reflect on our early understanding of medical science and recognize how far we have come, so it is that in future decades nutritional practitioners will reflect on today's pioneering approaches. Just as information in the field of information technology (IT) replaces itself every 18 months, so does that of nutrition science. Therefore, in this workbook, rather than stating absolutes we attempt primarily to speak from the experiences and outcomes of our practices.

In addition, there is a wide variance of opinions and approaches among nutritional practitioners — from the purists who insist on 100% organic to those who are concerned with calories only. In this workbook, we attempt to bring a practical approach to the person who is in the midst of considering a new direction with overall health and weight loss.

It is likely that your steps will be gradual, such as —
- eliminating carbonated beverages and artificial sweeteners.
- adding healthy fat into your daily diet such as olive oil and butter.
- counting carbohydrate intake per day, and other changes, over time that are acceptable to your lifestyle.

We hope that you will read and re-read this workbook several times in order to absorb the shifts in attitude and knowledge presented. These gradual changes in your perspective will facilitate those challenging habit patterns. We have found that once inner perspective is changed, it becomes easier to break the bad habit patterns.

The confusion over diets, such as high protein/low carbohydrate, low fat, low sugar, food-combining programs and so on, makes it very difficult for you to choose one that is right for you. In addition, these weight loss/gain cycles can contribute to many illnesses such as gall bladder disease, blood sugar disorders and food addictions.

It is also true that gaining and losing weight repeatedly results in more fat on the body and less lean muscle mass. In fact, every weight loss and weight gain cycle a person goes through usually results in a loss of muscle and a gain of fat. As many know, it can be difficult to build new muscle. So it is important to keep the muscles you have.

You may be gaining weight from eating too many *simple* carbohydrates, which in nutrition lingo translates into too much sugar. These simple carbohydrates convert immediately into blood sugar (glucose) creating abnormally high levels in the bloodstream. Every time you eat them, the body responds by producing insulin. Continuous insulin production is your enemy when trying to manage or lose weight.

Insulin's job is to remove the excess blood sugar from your bloodstream. Unfortunately, for most of us, the excess then gets stored into fat cells!

If you are eating these carbohydrates several times a day, you can be gaining weight every time you eat them. So you can see that the key to weight loss and weight management is to lower and manage carbohydrate levels, especially simple, fast-acting carbohydrates.

How sugars work in the body:
Simple sugars = Fast-acting = Glycemic = Blood sugar raising
Complex sugars = Slow-acting = Less glycemic = Blood sugar balancing

---

New research in biochemistry tells us that certain nutrients help us to manage blood sugar levels; therefore, our Plan addresses the need for nutritional supplements. We believe, and there is a lot of evidence to support, that we no longer get a proper balance of nutrients (vitamins, minerals, etc.) from diet alone. Farming techniques are less health supportive today than in the past, and many foods are transported over long distance from their source to the manufacturer. During this transport time, they continue to lose nutrients. Then the manufacturing process of foods, such as wheat and corn, can deplete up to 20 important vitamins and minerals. Cooking and freezing further diminishes nutrients.

The end result is that the typical American diet actually provides very little nourishment compared to foods produced by the farming and harvesting of years ago. We know of pre-packaged desserts that when placed on a plate and left uncovered for weeks or months, will not crumble, mold or decompose. In fact the bugs will not even eat them!

> **The manufacturing processes can be so vast that in the end one can hardly call it food!**

In a healthy state the body is capable of storing many vitamins, minerals and other essential compounds. It is like money in the bank and withdrawals are made on an as-needed basis. If the bank account is not being replenished, over time you end up with a zero balance. The crisis is even greater when your nutrient accounts are not being replenished daily. Initially the symptoms may be slight; however, the intensity and severity increases over time making you more vulnerable to illness and disease.

As if this were not bad enough, the typical western diet is high in what we call anti-nutrients. Many food companies add flavor enhancers, sugars and other additives to replace missing components lost in the manufacturing process. Anti-nutrients are like bank robbers who steal from your already waning account. It is no wonder we are operating on a deficit for most of our lives. Americans are the richest people in the world with access to the most food, and yet we suffer the highest levels of illness and disease. This is also becoming true of other technologically-advanced societies around the globe.

Finally, it is well known that today we are exposed to an increasing toxic environment which creates enormous stress on the body's immune system. Stress depletes all nutrients; therefore, you need more, not fewer, nutrients to fight back. We recommend you take daily a quality multi-vitamin and mineral product, and consider additional support from a stimulant free weight-loss formula (see *Appendix* for additional guidance).

Your Mind

Our *New Body-Mind-Spirit Approach to Weight Solutions* focuses upon the wholeness and interconnectedness of your thoughts, emotions, and physical body. Until recent years, the body and mind were considered to be completely separate. Scientific studies and research has followed, and continues to follow, that paradigm.

Especially as related to weight management, the medical establishment has long ignored one's mind and emotions as having anything to do with the physical body. In addition, childhood programming, decisions, and/or emotional experiences are not recognized as having any effect upon a person's eating patterns. Those of us in body-mind research know differently. The problem is that millions of people have tried to follow various and conflicting diet guidelines over the years with enormous frustration. When the negative mental or emotional energy rises, you are likely to sabotage yourself.

> **Changing negative eating habits and beginning weight loss
> will often trigger unconscious stored memories and emotions.
> This *rising* energy must be addressed for continued success.**

Reasons we hold on to excess body fat must be addressed. Without an understanding of the underlying *causes* for your sabotage, you may begin to feel discouraged at not being able to stay with a healthy eating program.

You may lose weight successfully, but gain it all back. You may begin to feel that permanent weight loss is hopeless and that there is no solution to the problem. This perception can increase the feeling of helplessness and low self-esteem related to your body. To make matters worse, everywhere you turn, the media promises over night miracles. Most people who have dieted over time fall into a downward spiral of discouragement mentally and emotionally.

In addition, you may not be aware that you might have caused damage to your physical body from continuous dieting. The good news is, however, that the body is always moving towards wellness, especially due to the physical improvements that can take place as a result of a healthier diet and lifestyle.

Our Plan will have you get in touch with your thoughts and emotions. In so doing you will begin to acknowledge, value, and give attention to your inner self. It will help to strengthen your resolve, and you will learn more about who you are!

Your Spirit

We believe that our body is the vessel for our *spirit*. Your spirit moves in and through this physical vessel with every breath that you take.

> **When your health is diminished, or your body is not operating at its optimum, it affects the energy that your spirit expresses in the world.**

The word spirit is also referred to as *life force*. In Hinduism, this life force is called prana; in China, it is called chi; and in Japan it is called ki. You can sense or feel a person's vitality and strength through his or her energy field. In a similar manner, we can sense a person's weakened energy field when he or she is ill, or health is diminishing.

Your spirit is carried by the form created by the joining of your father's sperm and your mother's egg. Your developing fetus carries the genealogy of your ancestors. This means that you may be predisposed to certain health issues according to those of your parents and grandparents. Until recently, genealogy was considered to be the primary determinant of your potential future health issues.

Nutrition and lifestyle choices deepen your inner work. The changes go beyond simply adjusting diet and increasing exercise. New research indicates that your nutrition and lifestyle choices will have a great impact upon the health of your body-mind-spirit. Our Plan will explore this as we encourage you to get in touch with your spirit, which we also refer to as your inner self.

Clients have confirmed our belief that *all* of your answers are within you! The examples we have used in this workbook are actual case histories. Names and occasional descriptions have been changed to protect privacy.

In considering our body-mind-spirit approach to weight management, we sincerely hope our Plan will bring greater success to your well being. We believe it will offer you the steps necessary to create a future with increased, rather than waning, health and vitality.

Through our experience, we have found that there is also a mind connection — what we think about our bodies is what we, in fact, create. According to Dr. Bruce Lipton, Ph.D., a cellular biologist at Stanford, of the four billion bits of information that our nervous system takes in every second, only about two thousand bits can be processed consciously. Therefore, more than 99% of your thoughts and emotions are unconscious to you. Your childhood memories, emotions, beliefs, attitudes and programming automatically move through your unconscious mind yet affect every aspect of your life.

Less understood in today's world is how your spirit is reflected in the physical body. You can either be diminishing or fueling your spirit. When your body, mind, and spirit are in alignment, you are heightened physically, mentally, and spiritually. When these three forms synchronize, your ability to succeed is certain. That is because you have a greater potential to experience profound joy in relationships, in careers, and in any other life goals.

We believe that the biggest misunderstanding in food choices today is in the area of low-fat diets and carbohydrates.

The first step to discover your way out of the weight loss maze is an awareness of basic nutrition and how it affects your success or failure. For example, an over emphasis on low fat food is fundamentally unhealthy and contributes to carbohydrate addictions and weight gain. When the body is deprived of healthy and essential fats, carbohydrate cravings result.

Before you begin the Plan, be sure to read the important pages following in the section called, "Your Body — Judith Speaks." This will give you a new perspective on fats and carbohydrate addiction.

Phase 1

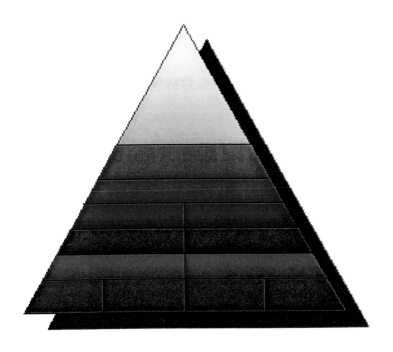

The Plan: Weeks 1~2
A Boost to your Metabolism,
Creating Discipline & Structure

The Plan

Δ

Phase 1: 2 Weeks
> A Boost to Your Metabolism, Creating Discipline & Structure

Phase 2: 4 Weeks
> Sustaining Metabolism, Strengthening Willpower

Phase 3: 6 Weeks
> Balancing Body, Mind and Spirit: A New Life Plan

Make a commitment to follow the Plan for at least 12 weeks.

**We have created this as a 12-week, or three month, Plan.
It takes the body an average of 90 days to shift its biochemistry.**

During the first two weeks, you will be asked to eat *no more than 30 grams of carbohydrates per day*. That means approximately 10% of your total daily calories will be from carbohydrates. In order to consume enough calories every day to support energy levels, you will need to *temporarily increase your intake of protein and fat*.

It is essential to *maintain a food diary* so you can monitor how you are doing. *We are lowering the amount of carbohydrates this much to provide a boost to your metabolism.* In other words, this shift in the ratio of carbohydrates to protein and fat sets up a biochemical opportunity to promote weight loss.

As we bring focus and clarity to cutting down the carbohydrates you eat daily, you may be shocked at the realization of how many carbohydrates (sugars) you consumed in the past. Obesity has become epidemic in our society as a result of eating so many carbohydrates, especially fast-acting carbohydrates, everyday.

It is critically important to remain on the Phase 1 Plan (30 carbohydrate grams per day) for the full two weeks. This allows an increase in biochemical metabolism to take place. It is also important to not remain on Phase 1 for much longer than two weeks. This is because the body needs at least 30% of total calories from carbohydrates to function optimally over the long term.

If you have been eating excessive carbohydrates over the years, you may have noticed the largest weight gain has been in the abdominal and waist area. This is how your body has reflected the biochemical imbalance of a carbohydrate addiction. It may have taken many years to manifest a gradually increasing weight gain in the mid-section of your body. It may take longer than you think to reverse this process. During the 90-day period, as you begin losing weight in your mid-section, see this as an excellent sign of progress. The slower the weight loss process, the more permanent your weight loss will be.

Our icon below will guide you toward correctly calculating your total intake of carbohydrates.

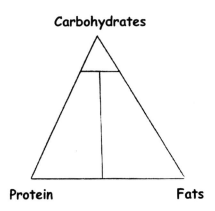

Overall Program

▲ **Eat at least three meals daily — no skipping meals.**
Skipping meals can kick your body into starvation mode. If your body thinks you
are starving, it will not allow weight to drop off.

▲ **Do not go below 20 grams of protein per meal.**
This is outlined further in the section, *Protein ~ Phase 1*. This is necessary to
maintain your lean muscle mass. The more lean muscle you have, the higher your
metabolism and the more fat you will burn.

▲ **Limit carbohydrates.**
This is outlined further in the section, *Carbohydrates ~ Phase 1*. You should begin
to notice the difference quickly in your energy, emotions, and physical body. If
you are exercising, you will notice changes more quickly.

▲ **Eat high quality fats at every meal.**
This is outlined further in the section, *Fats ~ Phase 1*. This will increase food
satisfaction, help you avoid carbohydrate cravings, and protect your heart.

▲ **Drink at least six glasses of water every day.**
Water enhances cellular function and this increases fat-burning efficiency.

▲ **Take all suggested supplements daily.**
This will help you avoid food cravings due to missing nutrients.
(For more information see *Nutritional Supplements* and the *Appendix*).

Daily Diary

▲ Keep track of all foods and beverages consumed in the Daily Diary (see page
26), and record carbohydrate calories and grams. It may be helpful to purchase a
reference book to aid you with measuring and recording calories and grams.

▲ Count and list only total carbohydrate grams and carbohydrate calories for the entire day. If you want to lose weight, this is the path to success! Later, as you become more comfortable with calculating all three of the food groups, you can begin to record fat and protein grams and calories as well.

▲ Keep track of nutrients in your Daily Dairy, or on a separate paper.

▲ Evaluate your inner emotional state and record it in the morning and before bed. Simplify with words, such as: anxious – nervous – excited – joyful – enthusiastic – angry – sad – worried – hopeful.

▲ Record your daily exercise.

▲ Record your daily total water intake.

▲ Enter your measurements and weight on the My Progress Report sheet (see page 31). Weigh yourself only once a week.

Prepare and Plan Ahead for Success

▲ Grocery shopping — take the list with you.

▲ Purchase enough spring or filtered water for the entire week. Don't forget lemons.

▲ Wash and cut up vegetables — put into sealed containers or baggies.

▲ Hard-boil eggs.

▲ Have easy protein available, such as unprocessed sliced turkey or lean beef, turkey burgers, turkey bacon, lean breakfast patties, and smoked salmon.

▲ Take the time to marinate and pre-cook chicken or fish for fast and easy meal preparation.

Daily Diary

We recommend copying this sheet or using plain paper for your Daily Diary.
(See Appendix for an example of Serena's Weekly Weigh-in Report).

Date:

Exercise: Mind/Spirit Activity:

Water: Δ Δ Δ Δ Δ Δ Δ (6 eight oz. glasses)
Nutrients: Δ Δ Δ
Protein: Δ Δ Δ   Fat/Nuts: Δ Δ Δ
Unlimited Vegetables: Δ Δ Δ   Grain/Limited Vegetables: Δ Δ
Fruits: Δ Δ

Breakfast   Calories   Grams: Carbs Protein Fat**
                           _____   ____   ____   ____
                           _____   ____   ____   ____

*Emotional Self: _____

Mid-morning Snack   Calories   Grams: Carbs Protein Fat**
                           _____   ____   ____   ____

Lunch   Calories   Grams: Carbs Protein Fat**
                           _____   ____   ____   ____
                           _____   ____   ____   ____
                           _____   ____   ____   ____

Emotional Self: _____

Mid-day Snack   Calories   Grams: <u>Carbs</u> <u>Protein</u> <u>Fat</u>**

_____   ____ ____ ____

Dinner   Calories   Grams: <u>Carbs</u> <u>Protein</u> <u>Fat</u>**

_____   ____ ____ ____
_____   ____ ____ ____
_____   ____ ____ ____

Emotional Self: _____

Slow Metabolizer 1,100 calories			Moderate Metabolizer 1,300 calories			Fast Metabolizer 1,500 calories		
Carbs	Protein	Fat	Carbs	Protein	Fat	Carbs	Protein	Fat
36g/ meal	28g/ meal	12g/ meal	43g/ meal	32g/ meal	14g/ meal	50g/ meal	37g/ meal	16g/ meal
110g/ day	83g/ day	36g/ day	130g/ day	98g/ day	43g/ day	150g/ day	112g/ day	50g/ day
440c/ day	330c/ day	330cal/ day	520c/ day	390c/ day	390c/ day	600c/ day	450c/ day	450c/ day

1 gram carbohydrates = 4 calories
1 gram protein = 4 calories
1 gram fat = 9 calories

_____

*Simplified descriptive words for emotional states include: peaceful, contented, joyful, fearful, angry, excited, irritated, agitated, nervous, anxious, etc.

**See _The Complete Book of Food Counts_ by Corinne T. Netzer.

Shopping List

Vegetables (unlimited)

Celery
Chives
Cucumbers
Lemons & Limes
Lettuce — dark, leafy greens
Mushrooms — portobello, shitake
Olives
Onions
Parsley & all fresh herbs
Peppers — all colors and types
Radish — red & white
Summer squash — yellow, zucchini
Tomatoes (fresh)

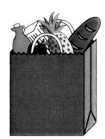

Vegetables (limited, 1 cup per meal)

Artichokes
Asparagus (8 spears)
Beans — green, wax or Italian
Bean sprouts
Broccoli
Cabbage
Cauliflower
Eggplant
Greens — collard, turnip, mustard, beef, kale, etc.
Kohlrabi
Leeks
Parsnips
Pea pods
Spinach
Sweet potatoes & Yams
Turnips

Water chestnuts
Winter squash & Pumpkin

Meat - Poultry - Fish

Beef

Cornish hen

Chicken

Duck

Lamb

Salmon, Orange roughie, Sea bass, Mackerel, Halibut, and other high-oil fish

Tuna, Haddock, Cod, Flounder, Sole, Sea trout, Red snapper, Scallops and other cold-water fish

Turkey bacon, Turkey sausage

Turkey breasts

Turkey breakfast patties, Ground turkey

Venison and other free-range meat

Eggs & Dairy

Chavrie goat cheese spread

Cottage or Ricotta cheese Hard cheese

Cream cheese   Soft cheese

Feta cheese

Hard cheese

Sour cream

Yogurt (plain only; full fat)

Eggs (free-range preferred)

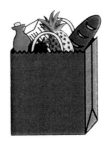

Fats

Avocado

Butter

Mayonnaise (Hain, Nayonnaise)

Olive oil (virgin)

Salad dressings (cold-pressed oils)

Nuts & Seeds

Almonds, cashews, pecans, walnuts,
   peanuts, pine nuts
Sunflower seeds, sesame seeds, flax seeds and pumpkin seeds

Fruits (low sugar)

Blueberries
Blackberries
Grapefruit
Raspberries
Strawberries
Tangerine, Orange

Beverages

Spring water, Mineral water, Fruit flavored sparkling water

Tomato juice (dilute with $\frac{1}{2}$ water)
Vegetable juice (dilute with $\frac{1}{2}$ water)
Herbal teas (hot or cold — sweeten with liquid Stevia if desired)
De-caf coffee (steam-processed decaf recommended)

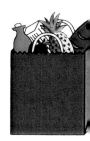

After Grocery Shopping, Save Time:

▲ Wash and cut-up vegetables; put in baggies.
▲ Hard-boil or devil eggs.
▲ Marinate chicken, turkey or fish; roast or grill ahead of time, if desired, for fast and easy meal preparation.
▲ Pan-fry turkey breakfast patties, turkey sausages or turkey burgers; warm up later in week as needed.
▲ Prepare "Better Butter" recipe. (see *Quick & Easy Recipes, Phase I*)
▲ Prepare soups, stews or stir-fries and refrigerate or freeze in small containers.

My Progress Report

Starting date: _____

Weight: _____

Measurements:
Bust/chest: _____
Waist: _____
Abdomen: _____
Hips: _____

After Phase 1:
Date: _____
Weight: _____

Measurements:
Bust/chest: _____
Waist: _____
Abdomen: _____
Hips: _____

After Phase 2:
Date: _____
Weight: _____

Measurements:
Bust/chest: _____
Waist: _____
Abdomen: _____
Hips: _____

After 9 weeks:

Date: _____

Weight: _____

Measurements:

Bust/chest: _____

Waist: _____

Abdomen: _____

Hips: _____

After 12 weeks:

Date: _____

Weight: _____

Measurements:

Bust/chest: _____

Waist: _____

Abdomen: _____

Hips: _____

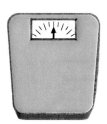

Carbohydrates - Phase 1

Weeks 1 and 2

Eat no more than 30 grams of carbohydrates per day.
After that period, in Phase 2, you will be able to increase your carbohydrate intake.

Eat two large salads per day made with dark green or red lettuce (romaine, radicchio, spinach, other green or red leaf), and an array of vegetables from the list below. Get a wide variety of vegetables over the course of the week.

If you suffer from diverticulosis, irritable bowel, Crohn's disease, or other gastrointestinal (GI) tract inflammatory-type ailments, cook all of your vegetables.

Unlimited: Eat any time
>   Beans — green, wax, or Italian
>   Celery
>   Chinese cabbage — green, white or red
>   Chives
>   Cucumbers
>   Lettuce — dark, leafy greens <u>only.</u>
>   (<u>Note:</u> iceberg lettuce does not contain some very important minerals)
>   Mushrooms — especially portobello, shitake and other exotic varieties
>   Onion — raw only
>   Parsley & all fresh herbs
>   Peppers — all colors and types
>   Radish —red & white
>   Spinach
>   Summer squash — yellow, zucchini
>   Tomatoes — fresh, and canned only with no sugar added

Limited: Up to 1 cup cooked, 2 cups raw, 1½ cups combined cooked and raw per day

        Artichokes
        Asparagus
        Bean sprouts (keep well rinsed)
        Broccoli
        Brussel sprouts
        Cauliflower
        Eggplant
        Greens — collard, turnip, mustard, etc.
        Kohlrabi
        Leeks
        Parsnips
        Pea pods
        Pumpkin
        Sweet potatoes & Yams
        Turnips
        Water chestnuts
        Winter squashes

Garnishes: Season to taste

        Chopped hardboiled egg
        Crumbled turkey bacon
        Grated cheese, Feta cheese, Goat cheese
        Nuts & seeds
        Olives

Making Vegetables More Fun!

Mother always said, "Eat your vegetables." Well, there is a reason for that. Vegetables are high in cancer-preventing nutrients such as antioxidants and other phyto (plant) compounds. Eating them encourages us to chew more. Chewing increases digestion and burns extra calories (10% per day or 150 extra burned calories with a 1,500 calorie per day diet). In addition, chewing keeps the entire GI tract, as well as the mouth, jaw and teeth, healthier.

Be Creative:

Δ Cold Veggie Salads
Garnish with any two of the following:
- 5–6 olives
- 2–3 Tbs. chopped nuts and/or seeds
- A crumbled hard-boiled egg
- 2 pieces of crumbled turkey bacon
- 1–2 Tbs. salad dressing, or olive oil and lemon
- 2 Tbs. grated Parmesan or Romano cheese
- 1 oz. Feta cheese

Δ Hot Veggie Salads   (1 c. steamed veggies and/or wilted greens)
Season with any two of the following:
- 1 Tbs. Butter or "Better Butter" (see *Quick & Easy Recipes, Phase 1*)
- 1–2 Tbs. salad dressing, or olive oil and lemon
- 2–3 Tbs. chopped nuts and/or seeds
- 4 tsp. olive oil and 1–2 tsp. Grey Poupon mustard, blended

Δ Stir Fry Veggies
Season with any two of the following:
- 1–2 Tbs. olive oil, or cold-pressed sesame seed oil, or
- 1-2 Tbs. "Better Butter"
- 2–3 Tbs. chopped nuts and/or seeds
- 1 oz. Feta cheese

My Working Journal

My favorite carbohydrates choices for Phase 1:

_____

_____

_____

_____

_____

_____

_____

_____

_____

_____

_____

_____

_____

_____

_____

_____

_____

_____

_____

_____

_____

_____

_____

_____

_____

_____

_____

_____

_____

_____

_____

_____

_____

Protein - Phase 1

Do not go below 20 grams of protein at every meal.
It is important to eat adequate levels of protein daily to maintain your lean muscle mass as you lose weight. In our experience, we have found that people do not consume enough protein at every meal rather than eating too much.

Note that pork is not listed as a protein source and should be eaten only occasionally, if at all. Research has found that eating pork creates negative changes to blood chemistry when blood samples are viewed through dark field microscopy. (In *Nourishing Traditions,* Dr. Olympia Pinto of Rio de Janeiro reported to author, Dr. Mary Enig, difficulties I finding patients for long term studies, because most participants drop out upon viewing their blood assays after consuming pork).

Remember that all foods contain some protein. You need not try and get all of your protein grams from meat alone (see *Protein Levels in Other Foods).*

Grams per day:

Meats: 3.5 ounces = 25–30 grams (approximately the size of a deck of cards)

Lean beef, lamb

Poultry: 5 ounces = 35–40 grams (approximately 1 large breast or 2 large drumsticks)

Chicken, Cornish hen, other poultry
Turkey breast, turkey bacon, turkey breakfast patties, turkey sausage, turkey burger
(Note: look for brands without nitrates, nitrites, other preservatives, or sugar)

Wild Game: 5 ounces = 35–40 grams

Duck, quail, venison, other free-range animals

Fish: 6 ounces fresh or frozen = 40–45 grams (If canned, read the label for total number of calories and grams)

Salmon, tuna, orange roughie, sea bass, herring, mackerel, red snapper, haddock, cod, flounder, sole and other cold-water fish

Cheese:
Hard cheese — all kinds: 6–7 grams protein per ounce
Soft cheese — e.g., sour cream, cream cheese, and other cheese spreads, cottage cheese, ricotta cheese: 3–6 grams protein per ounce

Note: Avoid low fat and no-fat dairy products as they are known to contain damaged (rancid) cholesterol molecules and are harmful to the body (see *Nourishing Traditions* by Sally Fallon and Mary Enig, Ph.D., or go to www.westonaprice.org).

Egg: 1 large egg = 6 grams protein

Vegetarian: Fake "meat" soy foods do not contain absorbable protein and are, therefore, not listed below as choices

Beans — ½ cup = 7–10 grams protein
Firm tofu — ½ cup = 10 grams protein
Tempeh, Natto — ½ cup = 16 grams protein

Protein Levels In Other Foods

The New Body-Mind-Spirit Approach to Weight Solutions recommends that you do not go below a minimum of 20 grams of protein per meal.

However, you do not need to get all of your protein grams from meat alone. Many people will become constipated, experience other digestive problems, or suffer from imbalances such as gout, if they eat too much animal protein. Remember that there is a varying amount of protein in many other foods, so add these to your grocery list as well.

If you are a vegetarian, it is just as important for you to get the recommended number of protein grams per meal. Some of our sickest clients are vegans or strict vegetarians who have extremely unhealthy (low) protein levels as measured by a comprehensive metabolic blood test. Low protein levels in the body can contribute to weakened immune function, reproductive problems, poor hair and nail quality, bone loss, skin conditions, blood sugar imbalances, carbohydrate cravings and more.

You will also note that we have not listed highly processed soy foods here as protein food choices. This is because we believe that foods such as soy burgers, soy hot dogs, fake soy meat and fake cheeses are just as unhealthy as any other highly processed food. In addition, due to the extreme processing techniques used, these foods do not provide absorbable protein to the consumer.

To make your job easier, we recommend that you purchase a food calorie and gram counter such as *The Complete Book of Food Counts* by Corinne T. Netzer, which can be found in most bookstores. We have used this book as a source.

Below is a sample list of protein grams in some non-meat foods:

Nuts:	Protein
Almonds, 1 oz.	5.9 g
Almond butter, 2 Tbs. (natural)	5 g
Cashews, 1 oz.	4.3 g
Peanut butter, 2 Tbs. (natural)	7.0 g
Peanuts, 1 oz.	8.0 g
Pecans, 1 oz.	2.5 g
Sesame seeds, ¼ c.	7 g
Sunflower seeds, ¼ c.	7 g
Tahini, 2 Tbs.	6 g
Walnuts, 1 oz.	2.5 g

Egg & Cheese:	
Egg, 1 whole	6 g
Blue cheese, ¼ c. crumbled	6 g
Chavrie spread, 2 Tbs.	3 g
Cheese, 1 oz. slice	5 g
Cottage cheese, ½ c.	13 g
Feta, 3 Tbs.	5 g
Goat cheese, 1 oz.	
Hard	8.7 g
Semi-soft	6.1 g
Soft	5.3 g
Hard cheese, 1 oz.	7 g

Veggies:	
Asparagus, 5 spears	2 g
Broccoli, 1 stalk	5 g
Cauliflower, 1/6 medium head	2 g
Mushrooms, 5 medium	3 g
Spinach, ¾ c. frozen	3 g

Beans:	
Most cooked beans, ½ c.	7–10 g

My Working Journal

My favorite protein choices for Phase 1:

_____
_____
_____
_____
_____
_____
_____
_____
_____
_____
_____
_____
_____
_____
_____
_____
_____
_____
_____
_____
_____
_____
_____
_____
_____
_____
_____
_____
_____
_____

Fats - Phase 1

Be sure to consume 14–16 grams of fat at each meal.
High-quality fats are important in order to avoid carbohydrate cravings. An enjoyable way to increase fat is to add cheese, which is listed with protein.

Avoid *low fat* and *no-fat* foods because they are extremely high in carbohydrates and/or sugars to compensate for the lack in taste.

It is preferable to eat *full-fat* dairy products. Biochemist Dr. Mary Enig discovered that 2%, 1%, and skim milk dairy products contain damaged (rancid) cholesterol. See www.westonaprice.org for more information.

You may use fats from the list below for flavor or add to cooking. Fat is a concentrated source of calories (9 calories per gram compared to 4 calories per gram for carbohydrates or protein).

Fat Choices:

Almond or walnut oil — do not heat (1 Tbs. = 14g)
 "Better-Butter" (1 stick butter, 7 Tbs. olive oil whisked and hardened in
  refrigerator; 1 Tbs. = 12.5 g average)
Butter — (1 Tbs. = 11 g)
 *Do not use margarine
Cream (1 Tbs. = 4.5 g)
Flaxseed oil — do not heat (1 Tbs. = 14 g)
Half & Half — (2 Tbs. = 3.5 g)
Mayonnaise (1 Tbs. = 11 g)
Olive oil — virgin preferred (1 Tbs. = 14 g)
Salad dressings — choose low or no carb (2 Tbs. = 16 g average)
Sesame seed oil (1 Tbs. = 14 g)

Seeds and nuts offer healthy fat choices. They also provide high fiber levels to the diet. Use as a garnish on salads, vegetables or other dishes, or use as a small snack ($\frac{1}{4}$ cup). Nut choices include:

Almonds
Cashews
Peanuts
Pecans
Pine nuts
Pumpkin seeds
Sesame seeds
Sunflower seeds
Walnuts

$\frac{1}{4}$ cup = 16 grams average

My Working Journal

My favorite healthy fat choices for Phase 1:

_____
_____
_____
_____
_____
_____
_____
_____
_____
_____
_____
_____
_____
_____
_____
_____
_____
_____
_____
_____
_____
_____
_____
_____
_____
_____
_____
_____
_____
_____
_____
_____
_____
_____

Fruits, Snacks & Beverages – Phase 1

During the first two weeks on our Body-Mind-Spirit Plan, fruits are limited due to their high carbohydrate level. During Phase 1, we recommend eating fruit as a treat *only if you have succeeded* in staying on the Plan. After each two-day period of following the Plan as designed, if you desire, you may choose from the following.

Limit to 10 grams
Fruit: Each indicated amount = 10 grams of carbohydrates

Apple — ½ medium
Avocado — ½ medium
Blackberries — ½ cup
Blueberries — ½ cup
Cherries — 10, fresh
Peach — 1 medium, fresh
Pear — ½ small
Plum — 1 medium, fresh
Raspberries — ½ cup
Strawberries — 1 cup

In order to cut down on the glycemic nature of fruit, we suggest having it with plain yogurt or 2 Tbs. of real cream (if whipped, use vanilla or cinnamon but no sugar).

Snacks

If you find yourself hungry between meals, choose from one of the following:

Plain yogurt with 1–2 Tbs. slivered almonds
Raw veggies and salsa
Raw veggies and almond butter dip
 • Blend 1 Tbs. almond butter with 2 Tbs. warm water
Deviled egg or hard-boiled egg
8–10 almonds, walnuts or pecans
Sardines in water or in mustard (1/3 of can only)
6–8 olives and l oz. hard cheese

Beverages

Flavored waters with zero carbohydrates and no artificial sweeteners
Club soda or mineral water with a twist of lemon or lime
Herbal teas (hot or iced)
Coffee or tea

Caffeine beverages tend to crash blood sugar levels leading to food cravings. They also keep insulin levels high making it more difficult to lose weight. It is best to limit coffee or black tea to 1 cup regular or water-processed decaf daily. We suggest herbal teas, hot or cold, throughout the day (de-caf coffee and de-caf black tea tends to contain residues of chemical that are used to remove the caffeine).

No Diet Sodas!   No Sugar-filled Sodas!   No Chemicalized Drinks!
Sodas are high in many different acids that tend to eat away at the stomach lining (consider the use of Cola to de-rust car engines). Sodas are high in sodium and potassium which can create bloating or fluid retention, and can unbalance electrolyte levels. These beverages also deplete calcium from the body. Diet

sodas have added chemical sweeteners which interfere with neurotransmitter function and can contribute to depression and moodiness.

For more information on the dangers of soft drinks, visit the following web link: http://westonaprice.org/modernfood/soft.html

 Alcohol is not recommended during the first 2 weeks. Alcoholic beverages are higher in calories than regular carbohydrates.

For example: 1 gram of regular carbohydrates = 4 calories; 1 gram of alcohol = 8 calories or twice as many!

Alcohol tends to crash blood sugar levels in many people, particularly those with blood sugar imbalances. This may occur in the middle of the night after having had one or two glasses of wine.

Blood sugar levels can drop below normal while asleep also due to consuming glycemic carbohydrates and chocolate. When this occurs, the adrenal glands will flood the blood stream with adrenaline. It is a primal response and our body's attempt to wake us up to eat in order to return blood sugar levels to normal.

If you wish to have a glass of wine later in the Plan, always drink it *with your meal, not on an empty stomach.* Many take sleeping pills for sleep problems, when monitoring blood sugar levels is a more natural solution.

Sample Meal Planner
for Phase 1

Breakfast

▲ Omelet with green peppers, onions, and fresh tomatoes. Add herbs to taste and sprinkle with 2 Tbs. shredded aged cheese.

▲ Turkey bacon, 1 serving (check food label for calories and grams) and plain yogurt with slivered almonds.

▲ Turkey sausage or turkey breakfast patties, 1 serving (check food label for calories and grams) with 1–2 poached or soft boiled eggs.

Lunch

▲ Grilled chicken breasts and dark green salad filled with unlimited vegetables. Garnish with $\frac{1}{8}$ c. nuts or seeds, or crumbled egg, olives, and 1 Tbs. olive oil and vinegar.

▲ Turkey burger with sliced fresh mushrooms and large dark green salad. Add garnish as above.

▲ Stir fried vegetables (1–2 Tbs. of olive oil) with finely sliced beef, chicken, shrimp, or tofu.

▲ Tuna mixed with $\frac{1}{2}$ c. cottage cheese or 1 Tbs. Mayo, served on bed of dark lettuce greens with cucumbers and tomatoes.

Dinner

▲ Broiled chicken served with asparagus and large dark green salad with feta cheese and unlimited vegetables with 1 Tbs. olive oil and balsamic vinegar or fresh lemon juice.

▲ Baked or poached salmon or other cold water fish, served with steamed pea pods tossed in butter and a large dark green salad with fresh tomatoes. Garnish with 2 Tbs. full-fat lemon yogurt and fresh cilantro, watercress or parsley.

▲ Roast turkey served with steamed Brussel sprouts tossed in butter and large dark green salad with 1 heaping Tbs. all natural dressing of choice.

Note: Mix and match any protein and vegetables from the list of recommended foods. Be creative, using herbs and spices, garlic and onion. Add all natural dried herb seasoning or garlic pepper. For salads, try *Newman's Own* or other cold-pressed oil dressings. Don't forget your healthy fat serving at every meal.

My Working Journal

For the first two weeks I need to focus on:

_____
_____
_____
_____
_____
_____
_____
_____
_____
_____
_____
_____
_____
_____
_____
_____
_____
_____
_____
_____
_____
_____
_____
_____
_____
_____
_____
_____
_____
_____
_____
_____
_____
_____

<u>Note</u>: Have I made my weekly meal plan? Which "Quick & Easy" foods can I keep on hand? Do I need to re-read the Plan?

Nutritional Supplements

Δ

Nutritional supplements are important components to the *Body-Mind Spirit Approach to Weight Solutions.* We believe it is critical to your success that you take *high quality* nutritional supplements daily, and do not overlook this aspect of the Plan. It may make the difference between success and failure.

If our body lacks just one vitamin, our appetite can be constantly stimulated to eat in an attempt to find that nutrient. When we turn to empty calories to fulfill that desire, our cravings are never satisfied. In addition, the underlying cause (nutritional depletion) never gets corrected. Properly tailored supplements can often provide the missing nutrients.

It is important to always work with a person who has been properly trained before developing a supplemental protocol for yourself. In not doing so, you may be taking nutrients or herbs unnecessarily, creating a biochemical imbalance in your system, and you may be choosing poor quality products.

Many supplements and herbal formulas on the market today contain unhealthy ingredients, or do not contain what the label states they do. Products to avoid are those that contain fillers such as sugar, yeast, starch, cellulose, salt and other unhealthy additives or preservatives. If you don't know which ingredients to avoid, research the manufacturer itself. Learn where they buy their ingredients, and what is contained in the *tableting base.* Many ingredients can present allergenic or toxic challenges to the system. Herbal formulas to prefer are those that say "standardized" on the label.

In addition, it is essential that the supplements you take can be absorbed and assimilated by your body. Products to look for are those that will dissolve in your stomach within 30 minutes. If they have not, then those nutrients may not be absorbed by your body — such supplements are a complete waste of your money. In order for an herbal weight-loss product to work optimally, it is best to add a high quality multi-vitamin and mineral product. This is to offset any deficiencies that might exist as a result of the lack of nutrients in your diet. Nutritional deficiencies may contribute to food cravings.

Eating May Not Provide Enough Nourishment

Some believe that you can get all necessary nutrients from a healthy diet. In Judith's practice this has not proved true. She has examined well over 500 comprehensive blood chemistries and found that typically clients are deficient in several nutrients. Persons can be particularly low in several of the B Vitamins, plus Magnesium, Calcium, Iron and Zinc. Results can also indicate low protein levels, indicating low protein intake or improper digestion and assimilation of the protein being eaten. In the latter, digestive enzyme supplements can be quite helpful.

It has been shown as early as the 1970's that Americans are malnourished. Congress mandated the *Health and Nutrition Examination Survey* to be run from May 1971 to June 1974. In this survey, the diets of 28,000 people were examined and, unfortunately, more than 60% showed at least one symptom of malnutrition (a lack of one or more nutrient).

> **USDA officials stated that if Americans merely improved their nutrition to RDA levels, 300,000 heart disease-related deaths and 150,000 cancer deaths could be prevented.**

Other studies, such as the *Ten-State Nutrition Survey*, have also confirmed vast nutritional deficiencies in the population. Sadly, the number of malnourished individuals has increased with each succeeding generation.

From our client base, we have observed that when people stop taking their suggested supplements, they may begin to notice increased cravings, re-gain the lost weight and experience a drop in energy levels. Even while taking supplements, some in weight-loss programs may take up to three months for *the first pounds to begin to shake off.* Most people give up too soon.

It is well worth the wait, however, even if it takes months or years to reach your desired goal. Your biochemistry speeds up your metabolism (i.e., the burning of calories) when you reduce carbohydrate intake and eliminate glycemic carbohydrates. When your body trusts that you are eating in a balanced way *for life,* not just for a short-lived or crash diet program, it will eventually allow weight loss to take place.

> **The biochemistry shifts when your body is consistently
> being provided the appropriate nutrients on a daily basis.
> This allows permanent weight loss to take place.**

Judith has searched several years to find a weight-loss aid that she could feel comfortable recommending. Many products on the market contain potentially dangerous stimulants, such as Ma Haung, Ephedra and its derivatives, or caffeine.

The weight-loss products we have used with success have been formulated using safe levels of certain herbs. These herbs stimulate the breakdown and use of fat for energy, can help to reset your metabolism and can build muscle mass. They will also increase your feeling of satiety (fullness after eating), and cleanse the body of excess water and toxins.

In order for an herbal weight-loss product to work optimally, it is best to take it in conjunction with a high quality multi-vitamin and mineral product. This is to offset any deficiencies that might exist as a result of the lack of nutrients in your diet. See *Appendix* for more information about nutritional supplements and herbal weight-loss products.

Nutrients Through the Skin

You may not be aware that your skin is a delivery system for nutrients. For example, the skin allows antioxidants and balancing hormones to enter the body. On the other hand, your skin can also absorb toxic ingredients such as those found in many personal care products today. It is important for optimal health to avoid cosmetics and personal care products that contain harmful ingredients, mineral oil, lanolin, waxes, synthetic dyes or fragrances, and animal by-products. We also suggest you choose pure skin care and make-up products that are botanically (herbally) based. This offers high levels of skin protecting antioxidants which can help ward off disease and slow down the aging process.

What Are Antioxidants?

Antioxidants are helpful compounds that slow down or reverse damage to cells and body tissue caused by *free radical activity*. Free radicals are molecules that form during normal cellular activity. They can also form during chronic infection and inflammation. Environmental factors can also increase free radical activity in the body such as ozone, the sun's rays, harmful ingredients in cleaning and personal care products, paint compounds, and X-rays. *Lipid radicals* are generated from consuming transfats or damaged cholesterol in highly processed food. Free radicals become even more dangerous when they multiply (in chain reactions).

Free radicals damage cells by attacking vulnerable targets inside the body, such as proteins, lipids, and DNA. The cell's genes take thousands of hits daily from free radicals. In a healthy body this damage can be reversed by units called repair enzymes. With increased exposure to free radical exposures, however, the repair enzymes themselves become damaged and are unable to keep up with the overload. This is when the body becomes vulnerable to illness and disease.

> **Many serious health conditions may be caused by free radical damage such as cancer, cardiovascular disease, cataracts, Alzheimer's and senility, arthritis, aging, lung disease and emphysema, high blood pressure, Parkinson's disease, and lowered immune system function.**

Antioxidants are best derived from foods: whole grains, wheat germ and nuts, fruits and vegetables, dark leafy greens, garlic and onions, as examples. There are many different antioxidants and they provide enormous benefits in a variety of ways. *We believe it is prudent to add a high-quality antioxidant formula to* your daily regime, and to place antioxidants on the skin via botanically-based cosmetics, in order to maximize protection against free radical pathology.

Some important antioxidants are:
- Vitamin A, Vitamin C, Vitamin E
- Carotenoids: Beta carotene, Lycopene, Lutein, Zeazanthin
- Flavanoids, Quercetin, Isoflavones
- Selenium, Zinc, Coenzyme Q, Alpha lipoic acid
- Catalase, Glutathione, Superoxide Dismutase (SOD)

The Incredible and Necessary Vitamin C

Biochemist Linus Pauling and others believe that at one time the human body was capable of manufacturing its own Vitamin C. But, due to a mutation of human DNA somewhere along the timeline of our existence, our bodies can no longer make it.

Almost all other species synthesize large quantities of Vitamin C when under stress or when they ingest carcinogens. When animals are injured, for example, they make higher levels of Vitamin C to aid in collagen and connective tissue repair.

Human bodies lack one of the four enzymes necessary to synthesize Vitamin C. Therefore, we need to consume it *daily* from fruits, vegetables, supplements, and from topical applications. This is the *only way* for humans to get enough Vitamin C, which provides maximum protection against environmental and drug exposures, chronic illness and disease.

Skin pH levels

In choosing personal care products, it is helpful to understand about skin pH. The skin's pH is approximately 5.5, which is slightly acidic and is called the *acid mantel*. The acid mantle is very important because it protects your body from bacterial invasion. It creates the proper environment for absorption of antioxidants and helps your skin avoid moisture losses. If your acid mantel is stripped away due to the use of unbalanced products, it can take three to seven hours to regenerate itself. *Products that are pH correct to your skin's normal pH level are the most effective way to get antioxidants into your body by way of your skin.*

Speaking of healthy skin...you have heard the saying that beauty comes from the inside. It happens to be true. If you are not eating a high level (3–4 servings per day) of fresh vegetables and 1–2 servings daily of fruit, you are not getting enough skin-protecting antioxidants from your diet and your skin will age faster. Pure water is also important to skin health. Water pushes out toxins and helps keep your skin from drying out. Also necessary for beautiful skin are the essential oils (EFA's) from fish and certain foods, such as olives, avocado, all vegetables, leafy greens, fresh nuts and seeds, natural nut butters, olive oil, and cold-pressed nut and seed oils.

Now that you have a greater understanding of the biochemical implications of unhealthy eating, and a better grasp of your nutritional needs, you are ready for the next step.

Healthy Nutritional Support to the Plan Includes:

- Multi Vitamin and Mineral Formula
- Digestive Enzyme Formula (broad-spectrum)
- Antioxidant Formula (if under high stress and toxic exposures)
- Herbal colon cleansing support
- Herbal Weight Loss Formula (non Ephedra, non-stimulant containing)

My Working Journal

My list of current supplements:

_____
_____
_____
_____
_____
_____
_____
_____
_____
_____
_____
_____
_____
_____
_____
_____
_____
_____
_____
_____
_____
_____
_____
_____
_____
_____
_____
_____
_____
_____
_____
_____
_____

<u>Note:</u> Do I take supplements? Are the ingredients from healthy sources? Do they contain additives or fillers? Have I worked with a properly trained practitioner to develop a protocol that is balanced to my biochemistry?

Physical Exercise
What is Your "Spirit Type"?

Before devising an exercise program for yourself, it is helpful to observe your natural inclination toward activity. For example, are you happier working out inside or outside? Do you prefer exercising with others or alone? Do you prefer to be entertained during exercise to make the time go by faster?

Would you describe yourself as a high-action or a slow-paced person? Answering questions such as these can help you visualize what type of body movement you tend toward and the environment in which you prefer to exercise.

Some of us are drawn to slow, rhythmic body motion, such as dance, tai chi and yoga. Others prefer intense aerobic workouts like power walking, running, rigorous bicycling, racket sports, and high-paced aerobics.

It helps to determine your workout *spirit type* beforehand. If your exercise program does not suit your spirit type, you will not adhere to it no matter how motivated you are when you start. Ideally, the best overall program would also include the opposite spirit-type workout once or twice a week, for a full body benefit.

For example, if you are a *slow-motion* spirit type, you might add one or two sessions per week of walking with lightweights for added aerobic benefit. Walking does not *pound* the way jogging or running does, and walking in a park or comparably inspiring environment can soothe your spirit. On the other hand, if you are a high-motion spirit type, you would benefit from slowing it down once or twice a week. Yoga and rhythmic stretching and dancing to your favorite music will relax overused, tense muscles.

Resistance-type exercise is critical to maintaining healthy bone density and avoiding bone loss. Therefore, if swimming, for example, is to be your primary exercise, be sure to add two or three weekly strength-training sessions to support bone health.

The basic safety rules are the same regardless of what mode of exercise you choose. Check with your doctor before engaging in any rigorous exercise program. Stretch thoroughly before and after your workout.

Dress properly when working out in severe weather, wear reflective clothing if out after dark, and remember to run or walk facing traffic. It is safer not to wear a headset while exercising outside because you will not hear danger approaching. Be sure to hydrate sufficiently before exercising, and rehydrate after.

Never begin an exercise program by over extending yourself. Proceed slowly, building up your strength, confidence and determination over time. Have fun. You are not training for the Olympics. If you can afford it, hire a personal trainer before beginning a weight-training program. If not, take advantage of most free assistance offered by gym staff before starting out. If you choose running as your primary workout, be sure to schedule weight training to strengthen and protect vulnerable joints.

My Working Journal

My favorite exercise routines are:

_____
_____
_____
_____
_____
_____
_____
_____
_____
_____
_____
_____
_____
_____
_____
_____
_____
_____
_____
_____
_____
_____
_____
_____
_____
_____
_____
_____
_____
_____
_____
_____

<u>Note:</u> What is my spirit type? Which days of the week can I exercise?

Quick and Easy Recipes – Phase 1

Better Butter

1 stick "real" butter
7 Tbs. virgin olive oil

▲ Put butter into a container and let it soften, or place in microwave for 10 seconds. Add olive oil and mix with mixer until well blended.
▲ Cover container and place in refrigerator where it will harden slightly but remain spreadable.
Use on steamed veggies or in stir-fries. This is a much healthier spread than others on the market today and easy to make!

Egg Frittata with Veggies

2 eggs
$\frac{1}{8}$ c. milk
2 tsp. olive oil
1 c. veggies, cut up for stir-fry

▲ Blend eggs and milk together and season mixture to taste. Warm oil in large skillet. Add vegetables and sauté until slightly tender, yet still crispy.
▲ Pour egg batter into vegetable mix and cook, covered, on low heat until mixture sets like a frittata. Check often and slightly lift edges of frittata to allow liquid egg mixture to drain to bottom of pan. Cover last few minutes to firm-up top layer.
▲ Or, place skillet in low oven (300°) for 5 minutes or more until slightly firm, but not overcooked. Eggs continue cooking after removing from heat. Serves 1.

Scrambled Eggs and Summer Squash

2 eggs
⅛ c. milk
2 tsp. olive oil
1 cup chopped onion
1 Tbs. Parmesan cheese
Summer squash and zucchini
Tomato salsa

▲ Blend eggs and milk together and season to taste. Warm oil up in large skillet. Add onion and squash and sauté only 2–3 minutes.
▲ Add egg batter to vegetable mixture and scramble together until slightly undercooked. Eggs continue cooking after removing from heat.
▲ Put on plate and sprinkle with cheese. Serve with a side of tomato salsa. Serves 1.

Moroccan Lamb Stew

1 Tbs. olive oil
1 large onion, chopped
2 lbs. lamb, trimmed and cut into 2" chunks
1 c. water
2 c. cut up sweet potatoes or winter squash, or a combination of both
1 c. pitted prunes (approximately 20) [3 prunes = approx. 10 grams of carbohydrates]
½ large lemon, seeded and cut into quarters
½ tsp. cinnamon
1 tsp. ground ginger
½ tsp. sea or Celtic salt
1 c. fresh cilantro, coarsely chopped
½ c. blanched almonds, toasted

▲ Heat oil in pressure cooker or large pot and sauté onion until lightly browned. Add remaining ingredients except almonds and stir to blend. Lock lid in place and over high heat bring to high pressure. Adjust heat to maintain high pressure and cook for 12 minutes. Let pressure drop naturally. Remove lid, tilting it away from you to allow steam to escape. If conventional pot is used, cook covered for 20 minutes or until lamb is thoroughly browned.

▲ Adjust seasonings to taste and transfer to a serving platter. Garnish with toasted almonds. Serves 4.

(Printed with permission from Sherry Krum, owner of The Wholesome Krum)

Barbecue Meal in a Bundle

2 pieces of fresh fish or boneless chicken breasts
1 sweet potato or yam
2 broccoli bunches, cut into chunks
½ Tbs. butter
Sea or Celtic salt, and ground pepper*
2 pieces of 12" foil

▲ Scrub, dry, and then cut sweet potato into chunks leaving peel on.
▲ Wash and pat dry fish or chicken. Place each piece of chicken or fish onto center of foil with edges of foil raised up to cup bundle.
▲ Add ½ of sweet potato and broccoli to each fish or chicken bundle.
▲ Divide butter in half and place a dollop of each onto bundle of food. Top with a sprinkling of salt and ground pepper. Add 2 Tbs. water to each bundle.
▲ Close up foil so it is tightly sealed. Place on pre-heated barbecue and cook 20 minutes for fish or 30 minutes for chicken. Be careful opening as hot steam will escape. Serves 2.
*Or use *Herb-A-Mare*, a sea salt and dried herbal seasoning found at health food stores.

Baked Fish and Hot Veggie Salad

Choice of fish: haddock, halibut, salmon, orange roughie, mahi-mahi, etc.
1 carrot stick, sliced
1 stalk broccoli, chopped
¾ c. red cabbage, rough chopped
¼ c. water
1 Tbs. olive oil
1 tsp. Dijon mustard
2 tsp. fresh lemon juice
1 Tbs. "Better Butter"
Sea salt, fresh or dried herbs and ground pepper

▲ Preheat oven to 350°, and melt 1 Tbs. "Better Butter" in 6 x 8 size baking dish. Be careful not to burn the butter.
▲ Remove baking dish from oven, add ¼ c. water and blend. Place fish in baking dish.
▲ Season one side of fish with sea salt, fresh or dried herbs and ground pepper.
▲ Place fish back into heated oven and bake approximately 6–10 minutes per side depending on thickness and density of fish.
▲ Steam carrots for 10 minutes, then add broccoli and cabbage and steam for another 6 minutes.
▲ In a measuring cup, blend olive oil, lemon juice and Dijon mustard and whisk together.
▲ Drain veggies, place in serving bowl and while hot, pour in the oil dressing. Toss lightly. Serves 2.

Grilled Vegetables Tossed with Balsamic Vinaigrette

1 medium eggplant, cut into thick slices
1 medium zucchini, quartered
1 medium yellow squash, quartered lengthwise
1 small red bell pepper, cut lengthwise into 6 strips

1 medium onion, cut into ¼ inch rounds
3 Tbs. olive oil
2–3 tsp. good quality balsamic vinegar
2 Tbs. fresh chopped basil
2/3 cup feta or goat cheese
Sea salt and ground pepper
Extra olive oil for drizzling on vegetables

▲ Preheat grill to medium heat. On a baking sheet, layer vegetables and drizzle with olive oil. Sprinkle with salt and pepper. Turn to coat.
▲ Place vegetables on grill and cook until tender and lightly browned, turning frequently. In a small bowl, mix the olive oil and balsamic vinegar. Put vegetables in large bowl, toss with vinaigrette. Sprinkle with basil and cheese and serve.
Note: this can be grilled on barbecue or roasted in the oven at 400 °.

Great Greens

Curried Mustard Greens:
1 bunch mustard greens or broccoli rabe (about 1 lb.)
2 Tbs. olive oil
3 large garlic cloves, thinly sliced
1 Tbs. curry powder
¼ tsp. sea salt or Celtic salt
¼ c. grated Parmesan cheese

▲ Cut off most of the thick stems of the greens. Wash well and place in 4 qt. pan with 2 cups water. Push leaves under water and simmer for 7–10 minutes, or until bright green and soft. Remove from pot and chop into bite-size pieces. Discard cooking water or save for soup broth, as it is very high in nutrients.
▲ In a 10-inch skillet, heat oil, add garlic and sauté until lightly browned. Add curry powder and mix well, then add salt. Add chopped greens and mix well; heat for 5 minutes, stirring often.
 ▲ Sprinkle Parmesan cheese over all, mix and serve.
(Printed with permission from Sherry Krum.)

Cuminy Greens:

1 tsp. olive oil
3 lb. greens (kale, chard, beet, spinach)
3 tsp. brown mustard seeds
3 tsp. cumin seeds
1–2 cloves minced garlic
¼ c. water
Pinch of sea salt or Celtic salt

▲ Heat oil in a heavy saucepan. Add mustard seeds, cumin seeds, and garlic. When seeds sputter, add greens, salt and water.
▲ Cover and simmer over low heat until greens are tender, about 15 minutes. (Printed with permission from Sherry Krum.)

Wilted Spinach with Olive Oil & Grated Cheese:

4 c. fresh spinach
2 Tbs. olive oil
¼ c. fresh Parmesan or Romano cheese
4 garlic cloves, sliced

▲ Rinse spinach. Heat garlic and olive oil in large skillet until warm (do not burn).
▲ Add spinach and continue tossing in oil until fully coated and slightly wilted.
▲ Remove from heat immediately, put in serving salad bowl and toss with cheese.
▲ Serve hot.

Weekly Soup

3–4 c. unlimited vegetables, chopped
2 tsp. seasoning: basil, bay leaf, parsley, ginger, onion, garlic, or mixed dried
   herbs
4 c. chicken, turkey, or vegetable broth
3 Tbs. olive oil
1 c. cooked chicken, turkey, or lean beef

▲ Sauté vegetables in olive oil with seasonings until lightly browned.
▲ Add broth and simmer 20 minutes.
▲ Add cooked poultry or meat and simmer another 5 minutes.
▲ Serve as main meal, or enjoy a cup before lunch or dinner.

Appetizer Soup Puree

This soup helps to flush the system. One cup eaten before a meal allows you to feel full. Wait 10 minutes before resuming your meal.

3–4 c. unlimited vegetables, chopped
4 c. water or broth
3 Tbs. olive oil
2 Tbs. cumin or coriander
2 Tbs. chopped fresh or dried parsley

▲ Place chopped vegetables, parsley and spices in water or broth. Bring to a boil then simmer for 20 minutes. Remove vegetables only and place them in a blender and puree until smooth. Return vegetables to the broth and stir until well blended. Pour into soup bowls and sprinkle with remaining parsley.

Cauliflower Pita

1 c. steamed cauliflower (per person)
$\frac{1}{2}$ Tbs. mayonnaise or Nayonnaise
$\frac{1}{4}$ tsp. Dijon mustard
$\frac{1}{4}$ tsp. Celtic or sea salt
1 tsp. chopped celery
1 Tsp. chopped onion
1 whole wheat or Ezekiel pita pocket

▲ Mash together cooked cauliflower, mayonnaise, mustard, salt, celery and onion.

▲ Spread cauliflower mix onto pita pocket. Gently place pocket in pre-heated toaster oven directly on rack. Bake at 425 ° until pita is browned. Garnish with grated red cabbage, or radicchio and carrots, if desired.

Jennifer's Vermontwitch

1 slice multi-grain or Ezekiel cinnamon raisin bead
1 apple, thinly sliced (Granny Smith is best)
1 slice cheddar cheese
2 oz. turkey, thinly sliced

▲ Top bread with cheddar cheese, turkey and apple slices. Place in toaster oven at 400 ° until apples are slightly golden. Serve with remaining apple slices.

Tummy Fillers

If you feel hungry during the day, replenish with water or drink a cup of herbal tea. You will be surprised how it may help to quell the hunger pangs.

Stuffed Celery Snack

Wash and cut celery in 5 inch pieces. Add one serving of your choice of filling:
Chavrie goat cheese spread
Almond butter
Natural peanut butter
Farmer's cheese

Favorite Nut Snacks

Choose your favorite from the following. By thoroughly chewing one nut at a time, into a liquid pulp, you will feel more satiated with this small snack.

10–12 almonds or hazelnuts
7–8 walnuts or pecan halves
18 unsalted, dry-roasted peanuts
2 Tbs. pistachios, sunflower, pumpkin or sesame seeds

Mandarin Orange Dessert Cream

1 envelope unflavored gelatin
$\frac{1}{2}$ c. orange juice (while fruit juice is not recommended on this Plan, the amount contained in this recipe is insignificant)
1 8-oz. can Mandarin oranges, water-packed
2 c. plain yogurt
$\frac{1}{2}$ tsp. ground cinnamon
$\frac{1}{2}$ tsp. vanilla

▲ Stir gelatin and orange juice in small sauce pan, mixing until softened. Add liquid from mandarin oranges and cook until gelatin is completely dissolved. Cool mixture. Stir in vanilla and yogurt and orange segments. Reserve a few segments for garnish. Mix well.
▲ Pour into four parfait glasses. Garnish each glass with remaining orange segments. Sprinkle with cinnamon and chill. Serves 4.

Falling Off the Wagon ~What to Do
Phase 1

We recognize that for various reasons you may not be able to be 100% accurate every day adhering to this Plan. The first two weeks are especially challenging. We encourage you to follow it with as much focused attention and care as possible. After all, that is why you chose to work with this program. Aside from weight loss, it is helping you to create:

- An eating program for life that will improve your health.
- Discipline to help you alleviate the inner struggle with weight management.
- A positive lifestyle for your body, mind, and spirit.

If you are not able to stay with *The New Body-Mind-Spirit Approach to Weight Solutions* Plan for one day (e.g., eating more carbohydrates than 30 grams), add one day to the end of the two-week period on Phase 1. In other words, continue to stay at 30 grams for each additional day you have *fallen off* the Plan.

Remember, however, that we do *not* recommend you stay at 30 grams for too much longer than a two-week period. We do not want 30 grams per day to become a regular way of eating, as it does not offer maximum health for the long term. For reduced carbohydrates to be most effective in terms of increasing your metabolism, it needs to be a short-burst eating program. Our Plan will have you increase carbohydrates to a higher level over two more phases.

We hope that the incentive to —
- give your metabolism the jolt that it needs for beginning weight loss; and
- increase carbohydrates later so you can move into Phase 2
will motivate you to stay on the program.

Reward Program for Good Diet and Exercise Behavior

One of the important components to successful weight loss and long term weight management is emotional — staying positive and not feeling abused. Our "inner child" often rises up demanding attention (e.g., "Why can't I have cookies/pie/candy [usually high-sugar foods]? Everyone else can.")

To insure that you are nurturing and giving attention to your inner child, learn to reward yourself with treats other than food. Here are a few suggestions to consider:

▲ Choose a week night that you are normally expected to cook dinner and take the night off. Tell your family or partner they are on their own, and plan a night of fun just for you.

▲ If you have a job where you can get away with it, take a couple of hours off in the afternoon and sneak into a movie matinee. Enjoy being a kid again.

▲ Spend some time this weekend with that novel that you've been anxious to read, with a cup of herbal tea; put your feet up and enjoy.

▲ Schedule a manicure or pedicure. You are learning to treat yourself and your entire body with positive attention.

This should get your creative juices going. Write down your own ideas and natural inclination toward fun and relaxing activities:

_____
_____
_____
_____
_____
_____
_____

Q & A for Phase 1

Δ

How long must I avoid potatoes, rice and bread?

This is a question we are often asked. These three foods are extremely glycemic and keep insulin levels high. As we have mentioned, it is very difficult, if not impossible, to initiate any weight loss when floating insulin levels are high. So in Phase 1 and Phase 2 we ask that you avoid all high glycemic foods. In Phase 3, you will be able to add back small amounts of these foods, balanced with a protein and/or healthy fat serving. At that point, we assume you will have lost some weight, your biochemistry will have begun to shift, and you can manage a few glycemic foods.

I've always thought popcorn was a great diet snack, but I don't see it on the list.

Popcorn comes from corn, one of the highest foods on the glycemic scale. Just think of corn syrup and other corn sweeteners provided to the food industry from processing corn. A way to lower the glycemic impact would be to sprinkle 1–2 Tbs. of grated cheese on popcorn. However, eating popcorn should be saved for Phase 3. Also, if you suffer from irritable bowel syndrome (IBS) or any other bowel-related illnesses, avoid corn and popcorn because they can be irritating to the lining of the GI (Gastro Intestinal) tract.

Since being on this Plan for a week, I have a dry mouth and bad breath. Why?

You are probably detoxifying sugars and other related substances. Every time we cut something out of our diet, the body starts shoveling out the excess it has been burdened with over the years. Keep drinking water and herbal teas, which might help with the bad taste; you can also use herbal lozenges. If you have access to a sauna, take one or two a week. If not, sweat baths three times a week (10–15 minutes) in your own tub with mineral salts will help speed up the release of toxins. Detoxifying-related symptoms might last for awhile and will eventually stop automatically. You may also notice skin eruptions on the face or other places on your body. This is usually temporary and should clear up in a few days or weeks. Remember, it is a good thing to clear toxins from the body.

Am I eating too much protein?

Over the long term, a person should consume 80 to 100 grams per day of protein from all foods (not just animal). This is calculated using a range of 1,100 to 1,500 calories per day. For example 1,100 calories x 30% = 330 calories from protein. Divide by 4 to get grams: 330 divided by 4 = 82 grams of protein per day. We don't believe anyone should go below 1,100 total calories per day because that becomes "dieting". After the diet, when the calorie consumption goes back to where it was before, weight usually increases.

Do you really mean we should eat full fat dairy products? Won't they make me fatter?

The reason not to consume dairy from low fat, 2%, 1% or skim milk is because they all contain powdered milk which has damaged (rancid) cholesterol molecules from the processing. These molecules cause free radical damage in the body which increases risk of cardiovascular disease and cancer significantly.

Some people are sensitive to dairy and cannot consume milk or cheese. If that is true for you, yet your symptoms are mild, you might try switching from cow-based dairy to goat, lamb or sheep dairy products. We have found that many of our clients can tolerate the dairy foods from these smaller animals. Also, in general, *cultured* dairy products (yogurt, cottage cheese, ricotta, feta, sour cream, kefir, etc.) cause fewer symptoms. This is because they have been somewhat *pre-digested* during the culturing process.

We know it is difficult to get that low-fat/no-fat mentality out of our inner tapes. However, to be disease free and optimally healthy, we need a minimum of 25 to 30% of total calories from healthy fats every day for:
- maximum cardio protection
- proper hormone balancing
- brain and neurotransmitter activity
- anti-inflammatory activity

- skin health, and
- the integrity of every single cell in the body.

When we don't get enough fat at every meal, we will crave carbohydrates — guaranteed. Experience with clients over many years has taught us that lack of proper fat intake creates many imbalances in the body.

Phase 2

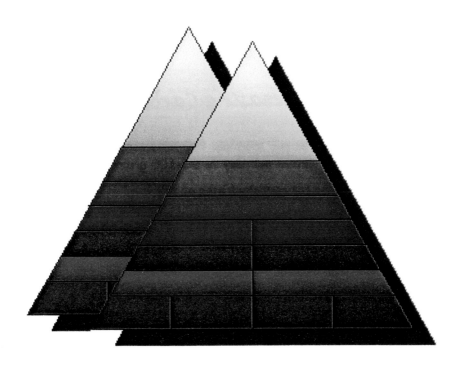

The Plan: Weeks 3~6
Sustaining Metabolism,
Strengthening Willpower

Changes to the Plan – Phase 2

Δ

Increasing Carbohydrates

At this juncture, you will increase the total number of all carbohydrates you eat daily from 30 grams per day to 90-100 grams per day.

You will continue to eat carbohydrates at this level — but no more — for the next four weeks.

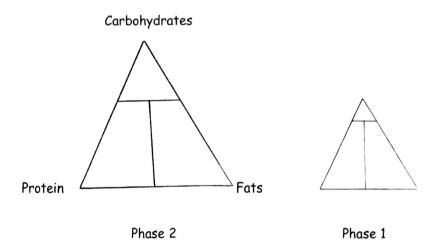

Phase 2   Phase 1

Remember to continue recording your calculations for carbohydrate grams in your Daily Diary. Your calculations can be approximate, but ought to remain as close as possible to the correct amounts. Some days you will be a bit higher and some days lower; it averages out.

You will notice that certain grains have been added to your list of carbohydrate selections. Some people are sensitive to grains, or as in the case of Crohn's or Celiac disease, may be severely allergic. This is often due to the gluten factor.

Gluten is the major *protein component* of wheat and other grass grains, such as rye, oats, barley and triticale, which contain similar proteins. If you are food sensitive or allergic it is best to avoid gluten-containing grains. Other grains such as rice, amaranth, quinoa, and corn belong to a different plant family, do not contain gluten, and can substitute for wheat and wheat flour (see *Appendix* for *Gluten Containing Grains*).

As an aside, it is interesting that gluten (grain protein) and casein (milk protein) are similar in their molecular structure. Often, if a person cannot properly digest gluten-containing grains, they may have similar problems digesting diary products due to the casein in milk. Many people mistakenly believe they are lactose intolerant when, in fact, they are casein intolerant. Of course, some people can be both lactose and casein intolerant. The one component of whole milk that fewer people seem to be sensitive or allergic to is the fat content. We have seen that lactose- and casein-sensitive clients commonly have no problem digesting 100% pure cream, which is entirely milk fat and does not contain lactose (milk sugars) or casein. You should choose *organic, free-range milk* whenever possible.

We recognize that it has been a disciplined two weeks in Phase 1. You've done a great job and we encourage you to continue to succeed with your goals.

Steps to Success:
Motivation – Commitment - Plan - Action

Success requires moving out of your comfort zone. It is important at this juncture to re-evaluate your personal motivation and commitment to growth and improved health.

You may have noticed that when you are highly motivated and committed to change, you become remarkably linked to resources as the Universe conspires to support your efforts. Teachers, books, articles and related information seem to find you. Philosophers remind us that when we are truly committed and take action, we can alter our physical and spiritual destiny.

Carbohydrate, Protein & Fat Choices

For your convenience, we have listed all three food groups again.

Unlimited Carbohydrates: *(Non-starchy vegetables)*

Beans — green, wax, or Italian
Celery
Chinese cabbage — green, white or red
Chives
Cucumbers
Lettuce — dark, leafy greens <u>only</u> (iceberg does not contain important minerals)
Mushrooms — especially portobello, shitake and other exotic varieties
Onion — raw only
Parsley & and all fresh herbs
Peppers — all colors and types
Radish — red & white
Spinach
Summer squash — yellow, zucchini
Tomatoes — fresh, and canned only with no sugar added

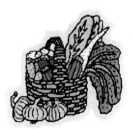

These vegetables have the lowest glycemic index, which means their sugars digest slowly and cause only a minimal rise in glucose (blood sugar) and insulin levels.

Limited Carbohydrates:

Up to 1 cup cooked, 2 cups raw, 1½ cups combined cooked & raw per day

Artichoke
Asparagus
Bean sprouts (keep well rinsed)
Broccoli
Brussel sprouts
Cauliflower
Eggplant
Greens — collard, turnip, mustard, etc.
Kohlrabi
Leeks
Parsnip, Turnip, Pumpkin
Pea pods
Sweet potatoes & Yams
Water chestnuts
Winter squashes

Fruit:

Limit to 20 grams per day. Each fruit indicated = 10 g of carbohydrates

Apple, ½ medium
Avocado, ½ medium
Blackberries or Blueberries, ½ cup
Cherries, 10 (fresh)
Grapefruit, Orange, Nectarine, ½ medium
Kiwi, 3 oz. small
Mango, sliced, ½ c. = 14 grams
Melon, 1/10 melon (7"x2")
Peach, 1 medium (fresh)
Pear, ½ small
Plum, 1 medium (fresh)
Strawberries, 1 cup

Grains:

Read label or check reference book for carbohydrate grams unless otherwise stated

Amaranth grain — ¼ cup dry = 31 grams

Barley, buckwheat groats, or millet — ¼ cup dry = 30–37 grams

Basmati or other brown rice, wild rice — ¼ cup dry = 33–38 grams

Bread — multi-grain or 100% whole wheat
  Sprouted grain bread
  Sour dough multi-grain bread

Bulgur (cracked wheat) — ¼ cup dry = 33 grams

Japanese-style brown rice crackers
  SAN-J Sesame Brown Rice Cracker — 5 crackers = 19 grams

Oatmeal (recommend 5 minute or slow-cooking; avoid instant) — ½ cup dry = 27 grams

Pasta — spelt, kamut, brown rice or whole wheat: 2 oz. uncooked = 37–44 grams

Pita pockets — sprouted grain or 100% whole wheat

Quinoa grain — ¼ cup dry = 19 grams

Ryvita, Finn Crisp or other European-style crackers

Uncle Sam's Cereal — 1 cup = 38 grams

WASA Crispbread Light Rye — 1 slice = 6 grams

Whole Food Baked Woven Wheat Crackers — 8 crackers = 25 grams

Whole wheat bread stick — 3 pieces = 12 grams

Whole wheat Crostini — 6 crostini = 23 grams

Maintain lower insulin levels by avoiding

glycemic carbohydrates (blood sugar raising).

Remember: high insulin levels = inability to lose weight or weight gain

For more information, see pages 144-145 on glycemic and

non-glycemic foods.

Reducing Protein and Stabilizing Fat Intake:

In Phase 1, you have been temporarily eating higher levels of protein and fat to offset the drastic cut in carbohydrate intake. These higher levels of intake are not recommended for longer than approximately two weeks, but are helpful in boosting your metabolism. Of course you need to eat, and it makes mathematical sense that if you cut back one food group, you must increase the other two in order to achieve the total calories per day that your body needs for energy and to function properly.

Protein:

Eat *a variety* of these protein foods and eat *at least* 20 grams of protein with every meal. Eat the specified amount of protein grams to maintain your lean body mass as you lose weight. This means eating at a minimum of 60 grams of protein every day.

Remember that all foods contain protein; do not try to get all of your protein grams from meat alone. You will also get protein from beans, dairy, nuts and eggs. If you haven't already, it may be helpful to purchase a reference book to help you count grams and calories. We recommend *The Complete Book of Food Counts* by Corinne T. Netzer. Here is a list of proteins to help get you started:

Meats:
(3.5 oz., about the size of a deck of cards = 25-30 g)
Lean beef, Lean lamb, Veal
<u>Note:</u> No processed luncheon meats, such as hot dogs, bologna or other processed deli meats. Always chose nitrate or preservative-free bacon.

Poultry:
(3.5 oz., about 1 breast or 2 drumsticks = 25-30 g)
Chicken, Cornish game hen
Turkey breast, turkey bacon, turkey breakfast patties, turkey sausage, turkey burger
<u>Note:</u> look for brands without nitrates or other preservatives, and no sugar.

Wild Game:
Duck, quail, venison, and other free-range meat

Fish :

(2-3 servings weekly)

3 oz. = 20–25 g (If canned, read label)

Salmon, Orange roughie, Sea bass, Mackerel, Halibut, and other high-oil fish

Tuna, Haddock, Cod, Flounder, Sole, Sea trout, Red snapper and other cold-water fish

Eggs:

(1 large egg = 6 g)

Scrambled, over-easy, soft or hard-boiled, poached, deviled

Cheese:

(Hard cheese — 6-7 g per oz. and Soft cheese = 3-6 g per oz.)

Hard cheese — all kinds, up to 2 oz. per serving

Soft cheese — sour cream, cream cheese and other cheese spreads, Farmer's cheese, 1 oz. per serving; and cottage cheese, ricotta cheese, ½ c. per serving.

<u>Note:</u> Avoid low fat and no-fat dairy products as they are known to contain damaged (rancid) cholesterol molecules, according to lipid biochemist, Dr. Mary Enig.

Vegetarian :

Fake "meat" soy foods do not contain absorbable protein and are, therefore, not listed as choices

Firm tofu — ½ c. = 10 g

Tempeh, Natto — ½ c. = 16 g

Beans — ½ c. = 7–10 g

Fats & Oils:

Remember, moderate amounts of high-quality, unprocessed fats and cold-pressed oils are important in order to avoid carbohydrate cravings. In addition, do not restrict natural sources of cholesterol or you may contribute to hormonal imbalances. Balance your fat/oil intake to approximately 60% from unsaturated oils (plant-based) and 40% saturated (animal-based).

You may use moderate amounts of fats or oils from the list below for flavor and in cooking. Fat is a concentrated source of calories (9 calories per gram as compared to 4 calories per gram for carbohydrates and protein).

Fat & Oil Choices:
For Cooking:
"Better Butter" (see *Quick & Easy Recipes, Phase 1*)
Butter — do not use margarine, commercial spreads or shortening
Olive oil — virgin oil preferred
Sesame seed oil — unroasted

On Salads or Hot Veggies:
Almond oil or walnut oil — do not heat
Flaxseed oil — do not heat
Roasted sesame seed oil
Salad dressings — choose cold-pressed oil with no carbohydrates

As Condiments:
Almond butter, tahini or natural peanut butter — 1 Tbs. per serving
Half & Half — 1–2 Tbs. per serving (subtract carbohydrates from daily total)
Mayonnaise — 1 Tbs. per serving
Whole Cream — 1–2 Tbs. per serving

Seeds & Nuts : *Use as a garnish or a small snack (¼c.)*
Almonds
Cashews
Peanuts
Pecans
Pine nut
Pumpkin seeds
Sesame seeds
Sunflower seeds
Walnuts

Behavior Modification

Now that you are becoming comfortable with the concepts of healthy eating, let's consider your behavior and habit patterns related to food.

During the 1960s, a new theory based upon behavior modification came into the field of weight control. The concept was that if a person learned to modify, or change, poor habit patterns related to eating behavior, he or she would lose weight naturally. During that period, Janet was an area director for The Diet Workshop, which was the first weight-loss organization to adopt behavior modification as an integral part of its program.

Working closely with this theory, Janet came to learn that the habitual eating patterns that one has will have an impact upon conscious or unconscious eating. For example, eating becomes very unconscious while reading a book or watching television. You aren't consciously aware of the quality and quantity of food that you are consuming. This lack of awareness adds to the confusion concerning an unexpected weight gain. It's easy to forget the potato chips and sodas consumed while reading, and think, "I've stayed on my diet. Why didn't I lose weight?"

We recommend that as you follow this eating Plan, you give attention to the following situations in order to change poor, often unconscious, eating habits. Good habit patterns are established when you are consciously alert to the food you are consuming.

Practice these techniques:
▲ Eat only in a proper dining setting.
  • Avoid eating in front of the TV, while riding or driving in a car, etc.
▲ Eat only as a solitary act.
  • Avoid eating or snacking while reading, watching television, or talking on the phone.
▲ Always sit down when you are eating, preferably at a table.
  • Avoid eating while standing.
▲ Eat slowly and consciously.
  • Pay attention to every bite of food that you put into your mouth.

- Chew your food at least 25 times before swallowing.
▲ Slow down your eating.
- Put your fork down between bites.
▲ Leave some food on your plate.
- Learn to shift the childhood messages that you may have heard, such as, "Don't be wasteful," or "Don't you know children are starving in……"

Practice these techniques one step at a time — or tackle them all at once. You know yourself best…and how easy or difficult these behavioral changes will be.

Quick & Easy Recipes – Phase 2

Breakfast Treat

1 slice Ezekiel sprouted grain bread (by *Food for Life*)
½ medium apple, cook in microwave and mash
1 tsp. cinnamon
½ c. cottage cheese

▲ Toast bread. Combine cottage cheese, cinnamon, and softened apple. Top bread with mixture. Broil until cheese is warm. Serve immediately.

Sesame Chicken

10 split chicken breasts, skinned and boned
¼ c. plain yogurt
1 Tbs. lemon pepper
2 tsp. basil
1 tsp. garlic, chopped
¼ c. sesame seeds

▲ Wash chicken and remove visible fat. Place chicken in a bowl and add yogurt, lemon pepper, basil, and garlic. Stir to mix well. Cover and refrigerate for at least 2 hours or overnight.
▲ With each piece of marinated chicken, dip into sesame seeds and place that side up in a baking disk that has been sprayed with olive oil. Cover and bake at 350° for 30 minutes, then uncover and broil for 5–10 minutes being careful not to burn the chicken pieces.

Parmesan Chicken

10 boneless chicken breasts, skinned and split; remove visible fat and wash
Brush each piece with olive oil and dip in mixture of:
  1 tsp. garlic granules
  ¼ c. Parmesan cheese
  2 Tbs. basil

▲ Place seasoned chicken in baking disk sprayed with olive oil. Bake uncovered in 375° oven until golden brown for about 15 minutes. When chicken is thoroughly cooked, top with sauce.

Sauce:
2 16-oz. cans whole tomatoes (no sugar added), blended
2 Tbs. oregano
2 tsp. basil
2 tsp. freshly grated garlic or 1 Tbs. garlic granules

▲ Sprinkle chicken with mixture of ½ c. Parmesan cheese, ½ c. grated mozzarella cheese and 2 Tbs. chopped parsley. Return to oven for 10–15 minutes until browned. Serves 10.

Turkey Meatballs

2 lbs. ground turkey
1/3 c. chopped parsley
¼ c. tamari
½ c. onion, finely chopped
1 tsp. powdered garlic

▲ In bowl, combine all ingredients until very well blended. Shape by hand into 1½ inch balls and place in oiled pan. Cover and bake at 350° for 35–40 minutes. Makes approximately 24 meatballs.

Lemon Chicken

1 large chicken, cut up and skinned
3 lemons, juiced
2 Tbs. olive oil
3 cloves garlic, chopped fine
Sea salt to taste

▲ Place chicken in baking dish. Mix oil, lemon juice, garlic and salt. Pour over chicken and let marinate overnight. Bake uncovered at 350° for 50–60 minutes.

Stir Fry

1 lb. boneless chicken (beef or lamb can also be used), thinly sliced
4 green onions, sliced
3 cloves garlic, chopped
1 c. bamboo shoots
3 Tbs. cashews
1 red pepper, sliced
1 c. water chestnuts
1 bok choy, sliced
2 Tbs. soy sauce
Black pepper to taste

▲ Heat olive oil in large sauté pan or wok. Add chicken and stir fry for 2 minutes. Set aside. In the hot pan, add red pepper, water chestnuts, bok choy, and soy sauce and stir fry for 1 minute. Add green onions, garlic, bamboo shoots, pepper, cashews, and chicken. Stir fry for 3 minutes, serve immediately. Makes 4–6 servings.

Roasted Green Beans

1–2 lbs. green beans, trimmed
1 each, small sweet red and yellow pepper, cut into strips
2 Tbs. "Better Butter"
¼ tsp. salt
¼ tsp. black pepper

▲ Heat oven to 400°. Cook beans in boiling water for 4 minutes. Drain. Toss beans, pepper strips, Better Butter, salt and pepper in roasting pan. Roast in oven 30 minutes, shaking pan occasionally until vegetables begin to brown.

Sautéed Spinach

2 Tbs. olive oil
2 garlic cloves, peeled
1 lb. fresh spinach leaves, washed and drained
Salt and freshly ground black pepper

▲ Sauté garlic for 5 minutes in olive oil until soft and brown. Add spinach and toss until each piece is coated and just wilted. Season with salt and pepper and serve immediately.

Spaghetti Squash

▲ Slice through skin of spaghetti squash several times. Simmer in boiling water for 30 minutes. Cool slightly; slice lengthwise and remove seeds. With a fork, pull strands of squash and place into a casserole dish sprayed lightly with olive oil. Top with 2 pats of "Better Butter" and 2 Tbs. Sucanat (unprocessed cane sugar). Bake approximately 20 minutes at 350 °.

Grilled Vegetables

zucchini, cut on diagonal into 2 inch strips
red onion, cut into 2 inch strips
red bell pepper, quartered and seeded
yellow bell pepper, quartered and seeded
cherry or grape tomatoes
eggplant, sliced into $\frac{1}{2}$ inch slices
olive oil
sea salt and ground pepper
$\frac{1}{2}$ c. balsamic vinegar
8 oz. feta cheese or soft goat cheese, crumbled

▲ Brush all vegetables with olive oil and season with salt and pepper. Place vegetables on the grill. Remove from grill as they become tender. Place vinegar in saucepan and reduce until thickened. Serve vegetables with tomatoes around the plate and crumbled feta or goat cheese over the top. Drizzle hot balsamic vinegar over the top and serve.

Eggplant

1 large eggplant
1 c. water with $\frac{1}{2}$ tsp. salt
1 medium onion, thinly sliced
2 medium tomatoes, sliced
1 c. mozzarella cheese
2 tsp. basil
1 tsp. garlic

▲ Wash and slice eggplant into 6 one-inch pieces.
▲ Dip each piece of eggplant into salted water and place on a cookie sheet that has been sprayed with olive oil.
▲ Top each with a slice of onion and bake at 350° for 20 minutes.
▲ Remove from oven and top each with a slice of tomato and cheese.

▲ Mix basil and garlic together and sprinkle on each stack.
▲ Place back into oven and bake for 10 more minutes. Serve immediately.
Serves 6.

Sprout Salad

$\frac{1}{2}$ c. mung bean sprouts
$\frac{1}{2}$ c. alfalfa sprouts
$\frac{1}{2}$ red cabbage, chopped
$\frac{1}{2}$ c. spinach, chopped
$\frac{1}{2}$ c. celery, sliced on diagonal
$\frac{1}{2}$ c. cauliflower, chopped
$\frac{1}{2}$ c. broccoli, chopped
$\frac{1}{2}$ c. red bell pepper, chopped
$\frac{1}{4}$ c. sunflower seeds

▲ Blend vegetables together.
▲ Serve with toasted sunflower seeds and a dressing of olive oil and vinegar or lemon.

Chinese Beef & Vegetable Salad

1 small cabbage, shredded
1 lb. green beans or Chinese long beans, trimmed
1 lb. sirloin, sliced very thin (freezing meat for 1 hour makes slicing easier)
2 Tbs. sesame seed oil
1 red pepper, cut into strips
1 large bok choy, sliced
3–5 cloves garlic, thinly sliced
1 Tbs. soy sauce
$\frac{1}{4}$ c. beef stock or water
$\frac{1}{4}$ c. sesame seeds

▲ Arrange cabbage on a large platter. Microwave beans for 6–8 minutes and set aside. Cook beef in oil over very high heat for 1 minute. Add red pepper, bok choy, and garlic and cook for 1 minute. Add soy sauce and water or stock and cook 1 more minute. Combine green beans and meat mixture and toss well. Spoon on top of cabbage and garnish with sesame seeds. Makes 4–6 servings.

Shish Kabobs

Marinade:
extra virgin olive oil
red wine vinegar
minced garlic
black pepper
herbs, as desired
▲ Marinate chicken, beef or lamb overnight.

Kabobs:
chicken, beef, or lamb
green peppers, cut into large chunks
yellow peppers, cut into large chunks
white or red onions, cut into large chunks
fresh cherry tomatoes

▲ Prepare meat on skewers, leaving space between chunks to cook better. We suggest grilling meat and vegetables separately on different skewers.
Note: If you put cherry tomatoes next to onions, the tomato will fall off from overcooking by the time the onion is done.

Yogurt Snack

4 oz. whole milk yogurt (no low fat or skim milk)
1/3 c. slivered almonds

▲ Mix well and enjoy for an afternoon pick-up.

Fruit Cup

1 c. fresh strawberries, sliced
1 c. fresh blueberries
1 medium kiwi, sliced fine

▲ Mix fruit and place in glass goblets.
▲ Top with a dollop of whipped cream or vanilla yogurt to serve.
One serving = ½ cup

Fruit & Protein Smoothie

2 scoops of whey protein powder
½ c. water
½ c. almond milk
4 oz. plain yogurt
¼ c. fresh or frozen blueberries or strawberries
1 tsp. vanilla
¼ tsp. cinnamon

▲ Place all ingredients in a blender and mix until frothy.

Falling Off the Wagon ~ What to Do
Phase 2

Δ

With the beginning success and accomplishments you achieved in Phase 1, it is our hope that you will continue to follow the Plan with discipline and attention. Nevertheless, if you fall off the wagon for one or two days, just add those days to the end of this four-week phase.

Generally speaking, lowering carbohydrates to such a great degree is the greatest challenge. Remember, we do *not* recommend that anyone remain at 90 grams of carbohydrates for much longer than four weeks.

This is a work in process during which you are becoming conscious of and improving your lifestyle choices and actions. Staying focused while on Phase 2 will accelerate you toward healthier eating for life, which should be a long-term goal.

Are you ready for your reward? Check it out...

Reward Program for Good Diet and Exercise Behavior

It is extremely important to reward yourself when you have had an excellent week and have met your goals. Rewarding your successes encourages and motivates you to carry on. Here are rewards to consider:

▲ After successfully avoiding desserts for several weeks, choose a day and treat yourself to a favorite dessert. Choose one that is healthier, such as a fruit-based dessert. As you learn to become more discriminating, you become more aware of ingredients. Make a big deal of the event — put on music, stretch out the time to enjoy, and congratulate yourself on a job well done thus far.

▲ If you can afford it, buy yourself that special something you have been looking at or thinking about. During the shopping trip, treat yourself to lunch or dinner at a favorite restaurant.

▲ Call that best friend you haven't talked to in ages. Have a long telephone catch-up or plan a lunch get-together.

▲ Schedule a facial or massage. Many people view these as luxuries when, in fact, they are necessary to a holistic physical and emotional maintenance program.

This should get your creative juices going. Write down some of your own ideas of ways to reward yourself:

_____

_____

_____

_____

_____

_____

_____

Q & A for Phase 2

Δ

How much will I lose?

During the first two weeks, you may have lost an initial amount of weight that exceeds what is typically advisable on a weekly basis. In spite of your excitement, it is not advisable to lose more than 1 to 1½ pounds per week, as measured by the scale, over the long term. If you stay with this Plan as a lifestyle change, over time this amount of weight loss can equal 30 to 75 pounds in a year. For *healthy* weight loss, you want to be thinking in terms of months and years, not days and weeks.

I did so well on Phase 1 that I'm afraid to increase carbohydrates. I don't want to gain weight.

As you can see from the visual below, the amount of carbohydrates increases slightly in Phase 2. However, to compensate, protein and fat intake decreases.

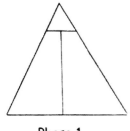
Phase 1

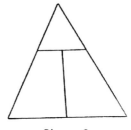
Phase 2

The visual indicates the importance of reducing fat and protein intake in order to offset the increase of carbohydrate consumption.

I've followed the Plan. Why haven't I lost more weight?

The scale is not the only measure of weight loss. Your clothes should feel a bit looser, especially around the waist and abdominal area. If you have been exercising, you may have muscle mass increase and muscle weighs more than fat, so your actual weight on the scale may not have shifted as much as you had hoped.

Don't give up! It may have taken many years to build up to your current weight, and it will take much longer than expected to lose it. For some people, it may take three to five years to reach their goal. The key is not to stop, but to remain committed to all three phases of the Plan in order to create a paradigm shift for the way you view nutrition. The healthiest way to lose weight is slowly, over time. When you consistently eat *healthy for life,* and daily provide all the necessary nutrients, the body will eventually allow weight loss to take place.

What if I plateau or begin to gain weight?

There could be several reasons for this to happen:

• You may have increased carbohydrates, but not reduced your daily protein and fat calories. Thus, you are consuming too many calories per day.

• You may have inadvertently increased calories by too much, and are not burning them off through increased exercise. For a week, count your total caloric intake, including carbohydrates, protein, and fats, so you can see how many calories you are consuming each day. You can then either reduce calories or increase exercise to offset those extra calories.

• You may have begun one or more prescription drugs, including hormone replacement or birth control pills, that may cause you to gain weight.

• If female, you are menstruating and are experiencing a temporary fluid weight gain. Try the herb, Dandelion Root, and consider using bio-identical progesterone cream on a monthly basis (see *Appendix* for resources). These are both natural diuretics.

• You may be bingeing due to carbohydrate cravings. If so, you may not be eating your 14 grams of healthy fat with every meal. Fat provides that feeling of satiety (hunger satisfaction) and must be consumed with every meal. However, be conscious of your fat grams because they can add up fast — more than twice as fast as the other two food groups.

• You may not be waiting ten minutes after a meal for feelings of hunger to disappear. It takes the various brain centers about ten minutes to register that you have eaten. Move away from the table and distract yourself for awhile, or enjoy a cup of tea. Hunger feelings *will* disappear.

• Are you consuming alcohol? If so, these calories will add quickly to your total caloric intake. Many people do not realize that the calories from alcohol are twice as high as the calories from carbohydrates...or eight calories per gram instead of four calories per gram. Alcohol excess can cause bloating or fluid weight gain....not to mention puffy eyes!

• Your body is just *re-setting* itself. Our bodies must make many physiological adjustments whenever the body size changes. It takes time for the body to re-set and literally reconstruct itself to adapt to any change in body weight. For example, it must reduce or increase the number of nerve endings, blood capillaries, and increase or decrease enzyme-producing cells and other body chemicals and tissue necessary to service higher or lower body mass. This happens to varying degrees every time depending on how much or how little weight gained or lost. So have some patience while this amazing process takes place.

Phase 3

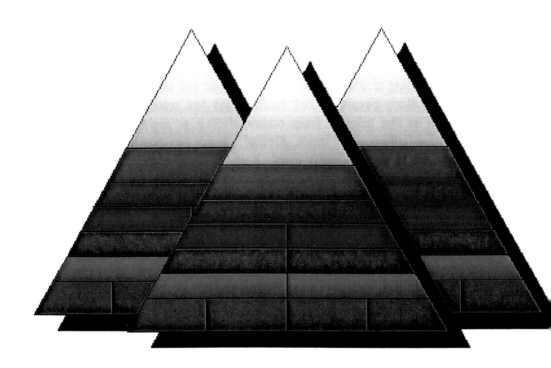

Balancing Body, Mind and Spirit:
A New Life Plan

Changes to the Plan - Phase 3

Δ

Your food choices in Phase 3 will be determined by whether or not you are at your goal weight. But first, a few words about setting realistic goals. Not everyone is meant to be a size 6. We all have different genetics which, based on our ancestry, predisposes us to certain body types. If we come from a family of full-figured women, it may be impossible to become *thin* and remain healthy.

There was a time in history when full-figured women were revered and exalted by artists. Even today, many cultures consider thin women unattractive and unhealthy. Also keep in mind that as we age, some additional weight can be a defense against the effects of a long-term illness. You may want to re-evaluate your goal weight based on more realistic thinking and desires.

In doing so, determine the total caloric intake that will assure comfortable weight maintenance. In the following examples, choose one formula that will help you continue losing weight or maintain your current weight. You can always go up or down in calories, and increase exercise, as you continue to reach your goal.

It is not healthy to eat less than 1,100 calories per day. The body's starvation defense system will kick in and not allow weight to be released. Once a predictable, continuous supply of calories can be depended upon by the defense system, it will relax and allow weight loss or weight maintenance to occur more easily. Survival responses force the body to defend against depletion of any kind.

Many diet books disagree on the percentage of carbohydrates to protein to fat. No one approach is cast in stone. *We have found the 40–30–30 approach to be the best answer for people who have struggled with carbohydrate addiction.*

Be sure you continue recording in your Daily Diary. You will now record all three food groups as to grams and calories consumed at each meal and snack. You will also total these for all three food groups, as well as total calories consumed every day.

Next, determine for yourself whether you are a slow metabolizer, moderate metabolizer, or fast metabolizer. This will aid you in maintaining your goal weight.

Are You a Slow, Moderate or Fast Metabolizer?

Most people who have difficulty losing weight are slow or moderate metabolizers. Alternatively, people who cannot gain weight are usually fast metabolizers.

Slow Metabolizer
1,100 calories

Carbohydrates	Protein	Fat
36 g per meal	28 g per meal	12 g per meal
10 g per day	83 g per day	36 g per day
440 cal per day	330 cal per day	330 cal per day

Moderate Metabolizer
1,300 calories

Carbohydrates	Protein	Fat
43 g per meal	32 g per meal	14 g per meal
130 g per day	98 g per day	43 g per day
520 cal per day	390 cal per day	390 cal per day

Fast Metabolizer
1,500 calories

Carbohydrates	Protein	Fat
50 g per meal	37 g per meal	16 g per meal
150 g per day	112 g per day	50 g per day
600 cal per day	450 cal per day	450 cal per day

*Remember: 1 gram of carbohydrates = 4 calories; 1 gram of protein = 4 calories; 1 gram of fat = 9 calories.

Daily Diary for Life

We recommend copying this sheet or using plain paper for your Daily Diary.

Date:

Exercise: Mind/Spirit Activity:

Water: Δ Δ Δ Δ Δ Δ Δ Δ (6 eight oz. glasses)
Nutrients: Δ Δ Δ
Protein: Δ Δ Δ   Fat/Nuts: Δ Δ Δ
Unlimited Vegetables: Δ Δ Δ   Grain/Limited Vegetables: Δ Δ
Fruits: Δ Δ

Breakfast

	Calories	Grams:	Carbs	Protein	Fat**
	_____		_____	_____	_____
	_____		_____	_____	_____

*Emotional Self: _____

Mid-morning Snack

	Calories	Grams:	Carbs	Protein	Fat**
	_____		_____	_____	_____

Lunch

	Calories	Grams:	Carbs	Protein	Fat**
	_____		_____	_____	_____
	_____		_____	_____	_____
	_____		_____	_____	_____

Emotional Self: _____

Mid-day Snack   Calories   Grams: <u>Carbs</u> <u>Protein</u> <u>Fat</u>**

——————   —— —— ——

Dinner   Calories   Grams: <u>Carbs</u> <u>Protein</u> <u>Fat</u>**

——————   —— —— ——
——————   —— —— ——
——————   —— —— ——

Emotional Self: _____

Slow Metabolizer 1,100 calories			Moderate Metabolizer 1,300 calories			Fast Metabolizer 1,500 calories		
Carbs	Protein	Fat	Carbs	Protein	Fat	Carbs	Protein	Fat
36g/ meal	28g/ meal	12g/ meal	43g/ meal	32g/ meal	14g/ meal	50g/ meal	37g/ meal	16g/ meal
110g/ day	83g/ day	36g/ day	130g/ day	98g/ day	43g/ day	150g/ day	112g/ day	50g/ day
440c/ day	330c/ day	330cal/ day	520c/ day	390c/ day	390c/ day	600c/ day	450c/ day	450c/ day

1 gram carbohydrates = 4 calories
1 gram protein = 4 calories
1 gram fat = 9 calories

————————————

*Simplified descriptive words for emotional states include: peaceful, contented, joyful, fearful, angry, excited, irritated, agitated, nervous, anxious, etc.

**See *The Complete Book of Food Counts* by Corinne T. Netzer.

Nutrition for Life - Phase 3

Δ

Congratulations! You have graduated to a new level of understanding. Even though a larger world of food choices may now be open to you, this is where knowledge, along with the discipline you have been practicing, pays off. In this section we will offer a more in-depth look at nutrition for life.

Whether you are a slow, moderate, or fast metabolizer, the proper ratio of carbohydrates, fats, and proteins at every meal determines successful weight management.

> **The fact is that most people gain back the weight they have lost, plus more. Will *you* beat the statistics? The answer lies in continuing the balance of foods that we have been teaching!**

You have been learning and practicing good nutrition throughout this Plan. It may help you stay with long-term, healthy eating if you know the reasons behind what works.

Most people can go on a diet and manage to loose weight, but fewer can maintain satisfactory weight levels. The key lies in balance and a deeper understanding of nutrition.

What is Nutrition?

Nutrition for life is health promoting while many diets can be health diminishing.

We define nutrition as:
- The useful totality of all we consume.
- The processes of absorption and assimilation.
- The availability of nutritive components for growth and repair to the cells.

The effectiveness of the above is determined by the *quality* of the nutrients we consume, the quality of the air we breathe, the quality of the water and beverages we drink, and what we apply to our skin.

You may be wondering what the difference is between diet and nutrition. Technically speaking, a diet is anything we consume on a regular basis. For example, some people live on a fast-food diet while others may exist on a one meal per day diet. One's diet may not necessarily be providing nutrition.

Many people feel as if they have been dieting to lose weight all their lives. "I am on a diet, so I must deprive myself." In reality, most weight-loss diets lack complete nutrition. As a result, the body craves nutrients. We are never really satisfied on a deprivation diet and eventually will binge. It is far healthier to consistently consume nutritious meals in a balanced way that does not leave us feeling deprived or empty.

It is also important to evaluate what you are putting on your skin because it can be absorbed into your body. Proper skin care is an important part of good nutrition. Wouldn't you prefer absorbing alive and beneficial antioxidants and other herbal, botanical compounds through the skin instead of dead and toxic chemicals, mineral and petroleum-based oils, synthetic dyes and alcohols? Check the ingredients in your personal care products, including your make-up.

Now let us look more closely at the components that make up nutrition.

Nutrients - Large and Small

Nutrients are divided into two categories: macro-nutrients and micro-nutrients. Macro-nutrients are the four food groups plus water and oxygen. Macro-nutrients are needed in large amounts.

Micro-nutrients are small components found inside the food groups, air, and water. They are used by your cells as precursors to create new body tissue, blood and other fluids, and as fuel to stimulate the creation process. They are microscopic units that are necessary for all cellular function. Micro-nutrients are needed in relatively small amounts.

Macro-nutrients	Micro-nutrients
Oxygen	Vitamins
Water	Minerals
Carbohydrates	Amino Acids
Protein	Essential Fatty Acids
Fats & Oils	Phyto (Plant) Compounds, and more

Oxygen - The Greatest Nutrient

The most important of all the nutrients required by your body is oxygen. You can go weeks without food and perhaps even days without water. Try going more than a few minutes without oxygen and its level of importance becomes frantically clear. To understand how vital oxygen is to your body, it is helpful to know a little bit about how your body utilizes it.

Oxygen is processed during the exchange of gases in your lungs called external respiration. It is continuously being demanded by every cell to fuel the process called internal respiration. The human body consists of many trillions of cells. Each cell requires oxygen to burn fuel nutrients for energy. Imagine just how deficient cellular activity can become within the brain and all tissue, organs, muscles, nerves, and elsewhere when these cells do not have adequate supplies of oxygen to support their needs. This is why daily exercise is so important!

Modern conveniences, as recent as the last 100 years, have eliminated 90% of the motion and exercise physical bodies used to have. It can be said that a sedentary lifestyle may have led to chronic oxygen starvation and, therefore, inferior cellular function. Given our physiological structure and needs, it makes sense that a daily infusion of nutrient oxygen is critical and essential for optimum health.

> **When you are tempted to ignore the importance of your daily walk, jog, or other physical activity, think of your cells suffocating from being deprived of their exercise, too.**

Water - What you don't know CAN hurt you

Many natural health practitioners believe that next to oxygen, pure, clean water may be the most important nutrient you can give yourself. As you age, your requirement for water can increase by as much as 10 to 15%. Most of our clients are dehydrated and do not drink nearly enough fresh, pure water daily, let alone increasing the amount. It is no wonder as we age our skin seemingly wrinkles and dries out right before our eyes.

In Judith's practice, people ask why they can't count other beverages consumed toward their daily quota of liquids.

> **Many of the liquids we drink — coffee, tea, soda, and alcohol — act as diuretics drawing fluid from the body tissues and systems rather than adding fluid to them.**

The effect of dehydration is similar to draining water from a car radiator and expecting the vehicle to run properly. In addition, many diuretics add polluting contaminants to your body's organs. Instead of flushing your system, they burden already dried out organs. Instead of quenching you, they corrupt your cells with sugary syrups, caffeine, and toxic chemical additives.

The average adult body measures 60 to 70% of its total weight in water. This figure is high because water, and the elements in water, are needed for myriads of bodily functions. You can lose up to two to three quarts of water each day through perspiration, urine, and bowel eliminations. You may not give much thought to your daily water requirements, but your body keeps track. Just a couple of days without water can cause serious harm, chronic illness and eventual death.

There is ongoing debate over the superiority of water sources such as filtered versus spring versus distilled. Most alternative practitioners believe that tap water is not a dependable source of healthy water. Many scientific studies support this theory. Consider for example, the Environmental Protection Agency (EPA) recently was not able to enforce water-safety standards for lack of money. It neglected to act on more than a *hundred thousand violations* in water systems serving thirty-seven million people.

If it were not enough that our municipal water poses such frightening hazards, other serious threats exist. These include ground water contamination, such as toxic chemical run off and heavy-metal presence from industrial, agricultural, and household run off and wastes. No one would argue that the quality of tap water has seriously declined in the last 60 years since many municipal water systems were first created.

Fortunately, there are ways to make tap water safer — some more convenient than others. Water can be boiled to kill parasites, aerated to release chlorine gases, and filtered using an in-home system. For best results, choose a quality home filtration system that has been approved by an independent lab; use that water for drinking, cooking, and rinsing foods. When traveling, buy bottled spring water to increase the quality of your drinking water on the road.

Many water experts recommend distilled water only for intermittent cleansing and flushing of body systems. Whatever filtration method you choose, making a thoughtful evaluation of the alternatives is one of the most important analyses you can make for your long-term health.

Carbohydrates ~ Energy Food

Carbohydrates are referred to as sugars and starches because that is their predominant make up as foods.

- Sugars and starches provide the primary fuel source for the body.
- By way of photosynthesis, the sun's energy is stored inside plant cells.
- Your body converts this stored plant fuel into stored energy (glucose).
- Complex carbohydrates provide indigestible bulk and fiber (cellulose).
- Fiber helps to maintain optimal blood sugar for consistent energy levels.
- Fiber helps to remove toxic matter from the body.

There is much debate, confusion and misunderstanding about how many carbohydrates one should eat in ratio to the other food groups.

The New Body-Mind-Spirit Approach recommends dietary intake of 40% from the Carbohydrate food group.

Your body converts carbohydrates into glucose which provides much of its energy needs. For explanation purposes, we place carbohydrates into two sub-categories: complex and simple. Complex carbohydrates are mostly whole plant foods found in their original, unaltered state, such as vegetables, fruits, beans, and whole grains. Whole grains have not been refined or enriched. For optimum health, these are the foods that should make up most of your dietary intake of carbohydrates.

As explained earlier, simple carbohydrates are primarily re-manufactured foods that, by way of a refining process designed to produce a longer shelf life, have had most of their nutrients and fiber removed. Such foods are denatured, devitalized versions of the balanced whole foods provided to us by Mother Nature. Since the 1950s, refined and enriched foods make up much of the American diet, such as enriched breads, pastas, cereals, snacks and most packaged and excessively processed consumables. In addition, these simple carbohydrates (simple sugars) plunge your blood sugar levels, making you hungry for more and feeding the vicious cycle of weight gain.

Like any other food, carbohydrates can convert to fat when we consume more than we can burn off in any 24-hour period. The excess is stored in adipose tissue for future energy demands.

What we have learned is that simple carbohydrates convert to fat far more quickly than complex carbohydrates. When eaten, these simple sugars combust into an immediate burst of *excessive* energy; in other words, more than we can immediately burn off. Consequently, the body takes the excess and, by increasing insulin levels, removes it from the blood stream and stores it inside your fat cells. Those of you who are expert dieters know how difficult it then becomes to burn off that stored fat!

The good news is that eating complex carbohydrates reduces your cravings for simple, fast-acting carbohydrates. Also, switching from simple to complex carbohydrates will lower your insulin levels and reduce your blood fat levels in a natural way. This is because complex carbohydrates contain the all-important fiber which is missing from simple carbohydrates. The presence of fiber slows down the surge of sugars into the blood stream. These sugars release slowly throughout the morning or afternoon, as we need the energy.

> **Fiber exerts a protective effect on the sugar-to-fat conversion.**
> **Processed, refined and enriched foods lack fiber.**

Overindulgence of simple, fast-acting carbohydrates leads to many disorders such as obesity, hypoglycemia, diabetes, adrenal burn-out, pancreatic deterioration, liver disorders, fibromyalgia and fatigue syndromes. In the carbohydrate category, choosing mostly complex-type carbohydrates in your daily diet supports optimum health over the long term.

Protein ~ Infrastructure

The protein you eat is broken down and re-configured to produce molecules called amino acids, the most common material in the body. Amino acid polymers are used to build components such as skin, blood, bone, muscles, hair, nails, and enzymes — catalysts that speed up chemical reactions of cells.

Children with growing bodies need more protein every day than fully grown adults. Think about this the next time you give your child cereal, bagels or any other glycemic carbohydrate breakfast! The first meal of the day should, as all others, contain a full serving of protein. This will provide the proper amino acids needed to feed the brain of you and your children.

Other important uses of protein in the body are:
- Construction and repair work.
- Production of white blood cells and antibodies.
- Production of blood serum proteins, collagen, elastin, and keratin.
- Builds muscle and other structural tissue.
- Production of neurotransmitters such as Serotonin, Dopamine and Norepinephrine.

The body does not use protein as a primary fuel source as it does glucose. Too much or too little protein can have harmful effects on the system. The Recommended Daily Allowance (RDA) for protein is 0.75 grams of protein per kilogram of body weight for adults.

Protein can be derived from a variety of foods including plant and animal sources. When plant protein is consumed, such as beans, it is important to combine the beans with a grain in order to supply all essential amino acids — also referred to as *complete protein*. Animal sources already offer complete protein.

**The New Body-Mind Spirit Approach recommends a
dietary intake of 30% per day from the Protein food group.**

We believe it is important for you to understand that the *quality* of your protein selections is a critical consideration. Much of the animal protein in the marketplace today has been altered from the way Mother Nature intended. While shopping, select hormone-free, antibiotic-free, additive-free, organically-raised, free-range meat and poultry whenever possible. Fortunately, there are a growing number of food stores that provide these healthier choices. If your store does not carry these, ask your grocer to make them available.

In the case of fish and seafood, it is healthiest to select those obtained from cold, clean water. For example, sea scallops are less contaminated than bay scallops. This is because the sea and ocean are less polluted than bays and harbors.

Did you know???
Meat, poultry, and some farm-raised fish can contain estrogen, growth hormones, antibiotics, pesticide residues, and preservatives, such as nitrates, sulfites, BHA, BHT, MSG, and HVP.

Fats ~ Building Walls in the Body

Many people seem to be as confused about fats and oils as they are about carbohydrates. A simple explanation and deeper understanding may go a long way toward protecting you from heart disease and related ailments.

Fats and oils are made up of *triglyceride molecules* and are classified as *lipids.* Lipids do not dissolve in water. Cholesterol is not a type of fat at all. However, because it also does not dissolve in water, it is classified as a lipid. Cholesterol is converted to steroid hormones and bile salts. Fats are usually solid and oils liquid at room temperature. Lipid stores in the body act as an energy reserve.

Fats are needed at every meal and are essential for achieving and maintaining optimal health. For example, lipid molecules provide impermeable membranes for structure and protection. Every cell in our body is surrounded by a membrane made up of phospholipids and cholesterol. This membrane provides a sort of wall around the cell so that cellular activity can remain segregated from unwanted outside interference. It is cholesterol that provides rigidity to cell membrane as it also enhances the function of many cell receptors. The quality of your cellular function determines the *biochemistry* of your body and is where, we believe, healing begins. Upgrade your cellular function and you will live a long healthy life.

The type of fat we consume is as important as how much we consume. Fats best for us are those that can be easily broken down by our body. These are natural, unprocessed, unaltered fat and oil sources. It may help to demystify the selecting of fats by analyzing them much in the same manner as our body does:
- Will they be dissolved and utilized by the body?
- Or will they just plug up the works?

Let us attempt to answer these questions by placing oils into two categories. In the first category are natural, unprocessed animal fats and properly extracted plant oils, such as those from nuts, seeds, and olives.

In the second category are all processed and refined oils, such as typical commercial oils sold in grocery stores today. Also included are all hydrogenated and partially-hydrogenated oils such as margarine, shortening, olestra and fake butter spreads. These are extremely high processed oils, called *transfats,* and they are added to most packaged foods. They are often referred to by food chemists as *plastic fats.* Do you want plastic clogging your system?

> **Biochemists have found that manufacturing processes deplete nutrients, make oils rancid, and destroy necessary enzymes. Manufacturing processes also modify the original molecular structure into codes that are no longer recognizable. They are unable to be broken down and used by the body.**

The single difference between these two categories gives us a clue as to how successfully the body can break them down and utilize them. Those in the first category are able to be dissolved and digested. The body recognizes these fat molecules and has the chemical capacity to put them to use.

On the other hand, those in the second category are unable to be dissolved because the body does not have the chemical code for breaking down the altered molecular structure. These fats have been changed from the way they were presented to us by Mother Nature and your body cannot use them.

The fat molecules have changed due to extreme heat, over-pasteurization, infiltration with hydrogen and preservatives, and have otherwise been made completely useless, and quite damaging, to the body. These altered fats are generally referred to as lipid peroxides; a form of free radical we know increases the risk of cardiovascular disease.

Seek out *cold-pressed* or *expeller-pressed oils* for use on salads and vegetables, such as olive oil, walnut oil, almond oil, and flaxseed oil. *Cook with fats and oils that are resistant to heat*, such as butter, olive oil, sesame seed oil, and coconut oil. Read all labels carefully to determine what type of oil you are consuming.

Now that you have a deeper understanding of the fat food group, you will pay closer attention to the type of fats and oils you consume. The fats you choose can make a big difference toward depleting or promoting health.

We would really like to recommend a higher intake than 30% of calories from fat, but have found that when we do so, people are consumed with disbelief and begin to panic. As a result, they default to their old ways of restricting some or all fat in their diets. They may unconsciously begin buying and consuming low-fat or no-fat food products, and unless quizzed, have no recollection of doing so. So for now, as a first step in awareness, we believe it is important to at least move you to the next level; that is from around 10 to 15% of daily fat intake to 30%. Even this is a major positive adjustment and the body can begin to repair itself from the years of damage caused by fat deficiencies.

The New Body-Mind-Spirit Approach recommends a dietary intake of 30% from the Fat food group.

Cholesterol Levels and Hormone Imbalance

According to women's health pioneer, Dr. John Lee, there are more than eighty known symptoms connected to hormone imbalance. Common symptoms can include:

sluggish thyroid, PMS, depression, mood swings, hair loss, osteoporosis, low libido, acne, breast cancer risk, premature development in girls, feminizing traits in males, fibrocystic breast disease, and insomnia — just to name a few.

Did You Know???
Cholesterol is connected to hormone imbalances.

Cholesterol is the precursor molecule that generates your reproductive hormones, such as estrogen, progesterone and testosterone. Many stress-related hormones are converted from progesterone. During times of unrelenting stress, the body's need for high levels of stress hormones can actually deplete your other hormone levels such as progesterone.

In our opinion, since the 1950's, the medical community and, therefore, the general public has been over focused on estrogen when we should have been observing and monitoring an equally important hormone, progesterone. Progesterone has many uses in the body. It uses fat for energy and is a natural diuretic and antidepressant. It also assists thyroid hormone action, restores normal sleep patterns and sex drive. Other hormones that can become depleted are adrenal hormones, DHEA, and testosterone.

Did You Know???
Studies show that 50% of women in America are deficient in progesterone by the age of 34.

So you can see that a cholesterol deficiency can have many implications in your body. When you restrict cholesterol or saturated fat in your diet, you may be pushing your body to manufacture more in order to offset the imbalance. The body needs cholesterol to maintain a healthy level of all reproductive and stress-related hormones. Avoiding cholesterol can inadvertently create deficiencies in many hormone levels.

We believe that vegetarians need to pay close attention to this information. If you are a vegan or vegetarian and wish to avoid meat, poultry and fish, you would be wise to consume daily eggs, butter, cheese, yogurt and other dairy products. This will help offset the missing fat and other nutrients one usually gets from animal food. Unfortunately, we have seen many vegetarians suffer needlessly from irregular or no menses, recurring miscarriages, and unhealthy births, much of which stems from a lack of adequate fat in the diet.

If your cholesterol levels are high, it may be worthwhile to discover the underlying cause before jumping immediately to the pharmaceutical approach. Your body may be keeping levels high in order to offset a hormonal imbalance due to stress or a saturated fat deficiency. According to Dr. Mary Enig's research, high cholesterol levels may also result from chronic low thyroid function. In many cases, correcting the underlying imbalance can lower cholesterol naturally.

As you can see, having a cholesterol imbalance is much more complicated than can be resolved by simply taking a prescription drug. We emphasize that you need to undertake personal research if these are issues for you. To help get you started, we recommend the following web sites: www.JohnLeeMD.com and www.westonaprice.org. See the *Appendix* for an in-depth *Resource* list.

Micro-Nutrients ~ Vitamins, Minerals and Plant Compounds

Micro-nutrients are nutritional units that nourish your body, such as vitamins, minerals, antioxidants and other phyto (plant) compounds, amino acids, and essential fatty acids. They are needed in only small or trace amounts. Healthy bodies manufacture and store some micro-nutrients, but many of them are required daily from dietary sources.

The RDA was established many years ago in order to avoid the possibility of illness or disease from a nutrient deficiency. We believe the RDA is the *bare minimum* of nutrients required to discourage illness and disease. It does not account for what is necessary to achieve optimal rather than borderline health. Modern science takes nutrient supplementation to a new dimension, making available successful therapies for the treatment and prevention of disease.

> **Cutting-edge research scientists and practitioners working in a new field called *orthomolecular medicine* have discovered that many illnesses and diseases are caused by nutritional deficiencies.**

Improving your diet, eliminating junk foods, and adding missing nutrients can correct the chemical imbalances of many illnesses. The theory of biochemical imbalance is based on the assumption that all of our biological interactions with food, water and air are an important part of good health. This is dependant upon the quality and proper balance of all nutrients.

The *correct* amount differs for each human body due to biochemical individuality. Also, nutrient requirements may vary from week to week and season to season, depending on fluctuating health. Because this topic is so vast and confusing, any decision to supplement beyond average recommended amounts should be made only with the help of a knowledgeable advisor.

> **It is important for patients who are taking prescription drugs to seek the advice of his or her physician.**
> **Some supplements should not be taken with certain drugs.**

Your cells could not function without a proper balance of nutrients. Cells are a busy flurry of whirring activity every second of every day during your entire life. Each and every cell in the body is a miniature chemistry factory that calls upon thousands of nutritional compounds to continually operate. These components are assimilated from food, air, water and other beverages which are converted into new molecules and compounds as necessary and become quintessential building blocks of your body.

The quality and the availability of these compounds to the cells pre-determines the quality, function, and vitality of the resulting structure of all of your body's systems. In other words, the quality and completeness of the nutrient base of raw ingredients you provide to your cells daily will give you back a healthy or unhealthy body structure.

> We borrow a phrase from the computer industry —
> *Garbage in, Garbage out.*

Anti-Nutrients ~ *Nutrient Robbers*

The term, anti-nutrient, refers to certain food or lifestyle choices that steal important nutrients from your body. Anti-nutrients should be avoided. Many are listed below.

> **Anti-nutrients can cause serious deficiencies in your body.**

Table Sugar:
- Depletes vitamin and mineral stores, especially vitamins B and C, and minerals magnesium and chromium.
- Fluctuates certain hormone levels aggravating menstrual problems.
- Creates extremes in blood-sugar levels.
- Severely damages your endocrine glands (e.g., adrenals, pancreas).
- Triggers hot flashes.
- Inhibits calcium absorption contributing to osteoporosis.
- Is addictive and added to most packaged foods.
- Is linked to obesity, digestive disturbances, tooth decay, diabetes, chronic fatigue, fibromyalgia and more.
- Increases blood fat levels making us fatter.
- Increases vulnerability to urinary tract infections.

We recommend natural sweeteners in small amounts, such as honey, real maple syrup, rice syrup, date sugar, Sucanat, and Stevia. (<u>Note</u>: Stevia, a plant-derived sweetener, is excellent for diabetics or carbohydrate addicts).

The Wisdom of Nature:
While vacationing with her husband, Judith observed this wisdom in action. Enjoying breakfast in an open-air restaurant, both she and her husband watched an amazing act of bird discernment on the part of a starling. On a nearby table were a variety of natural and artificial sweeteners. They included: packets of

white table sugar, Equal, Sweet 'N Low, and Sugar in the Raw. The bird landed near the packets and cautiously, with its beak, selected the least processed sweetener...The Sugar in the Raw.

Commercial Table Salt ~ Sodium Chloride

Salt comes from the sea and is a balanced source for your body's need for minerals. The ratio of minerals in sea water is similar to the ratio of minerals in body fluids. Commercial salt has been through so many processing steps that the result contains an unbalanced level of mineral salts: too high in sodium and chloride levels, and too low in other necessary minerals.

Did You Know???
The daily need for salt is between 1 and 3 grams per day.
The average American consumes 6 to 20 grams per day.

We believe the list of imbalances below result from the consumption of refined, commercial salt. Commercial table salt —

♦ raises the blood pressure, increasing the risk of heart and kidney disease.
♦ adds unwanted weight by stimulating water retention, and prevents loss of fat.
♦ triggers hot flashes and promotes loss of calcium from bones.
♦ increases and aggravates PMS symptoms.
♦ is added to processed and manufactured food to increase shelf life.

We recommend Celtic salt or minimally processed sea salt. Unprocessed mineral salts from the sea provide the body with an excellent source of minerals including properly balanced electrolytes. Electrolytes help regulate acid-base balance to maintain the correct pH of body fluids and skin, are necessary for maintaining normal blood pressure levels, and for normal function of the brain, heart and lungs.

Caffeine:

Caffeine stimulates the adrenals to produce adrenaline. In response, your body increases heart rate, stimulates your nervous system, increase stomach acid production and raises, then crashes, your blood sugar levels. We suggest you either avoid caffeine, or limit intake to no more than one cup per day; always drink it with a meal rather than on an empty stomach to minimize the symptoms.

Excessive caffeine —
+ depletes vitamin C and B-complex, especially thiamin — vitamin B-1; and minerals calcium, potassium and zinc due to its diuretic effects.
+ aggravates symptoms of fibrocystic breast disease.
+ constricts blood vessels surrounding the brain.
+ increases pressure to the eyeballs (glaucoma patients take note).
+ over-stimulates the central nervous system, speeding up the heart.
+ increases insulin response, which stimulates the appetite and raises blood sugar levels to an unnatural high followed by a blood sugar crash.

If you are sensitive, consider switching to herbal teas or coffee substitutes.

Alcohol:
We recommend that alcohol be limited to an occasional glass of wine or beer with a meal. The apparent benefits decline after more than one or two drinks. Pregnant women should eliminate alcohol for the duration of the pregnancy.

Excessive alcohol consumption —
+ inhibits platelet formation used to produce blood clots.
+ depletes vitamin B-complex, C, and A; and minerals such as magnesium, potassium, and zinc.
+ impairs calcium absorption, possibly affecting the liver's ability to activate vitamin D, increasing osteoporosis risk.
+ is highly addictive to some people and increases the risk of diabetes, heart disease and cancer.
+ damages kidneys, pancreas and liver when over consumed.
+ can aggravate high blood pressure symptoms.
+ provides surplus calories.

Smoking:
+ is considered the largest cause of premature death and ill health for all American men and women.

- depletes vitamins A, C and E, and many minerals.
- brings on an earlier menopause and intensifies hot flashes.
- increases facial wrinkling, especially around the mouth.
- can ruin a perfectly good face-lift!

Skin Care Products & Cosmetics:

Certain skin and personal care products can be considered anti-nutrients. Carefully check product ingredients listed on the packaging before using. Avoid products containing synthetic dyes and fragrances. Organic products may develop virulent molds or become rancid; preservatives are needed to avoid this. However choose products with low levels of preservatives. Keep preservatives below 1% in ratio to the total volume of ingredients.

- Heated and rancid oils contained in cosmetics can deplete liver function and accelerate the visible signs of aging on the skin.
- Certain alcohols alter the important acid mantel of the skin which fights bacteria and helps maintain healthy immune function.
- Mineral oil is seen by some cosmetic scientists as the No. 2 cause of aging, after the sun, and because it is a *xeno* estrogen can contribute to hormonal imbalances.
- Mineral oil, animal ingredients, lanolin and waxes can clog pores, interfering with the absorption of moisture and the release of toxins through the skin.

Trans Fats:

- Accelerate arteriosclerosis and other degenerative diseases by clogging the arterial system.
- Interfere with normal cell membrane structure and function, and block healthy fats (natural fats and oils).
- Block production of prostaglandins — hormone-like compounds that regulate every human function at the molecular level.
- Are devoid of nutrients essential for healthy heart function.
- Might magnify the carcinogenic effect of some chemicals.

The Wisdom of Nature:

Dr. Mary Enig tells of an experiment she conducted during one cold winter. On a window ledge she placed three containers filled with 1) margarine, 2) butter, and 3) cheese. Throughout the winter the birds visited regularly to feed from the butter and cheese. During the entire winter, they never touched the container filled with margarine.

Because of their convenience, anti-nutrients make tempting choices. We recognize that these categories may already be part of your lifestyle. We present this dark side of anti-nutrients not to frighten and overwhelm you, but because we believe that knowledge is power. Only you have the power to improve your health.

While it is important to avoid anti-nutrients, we know that change is a step-by-step process. It will take time to gradually make healthier choices and that is okay. Knowledge of nutrition can be a powerful motivator for weaning ourselves from unhealthy foods.

Make a concerted effort to avoid anti-nutrients on a daily basis.

The more you transition away from nutrient robbers toward whole, natural foods, the sooner you will begin to experience the benefits of balanced weight and extraordinarily good health. Remember every change we make, whether physical, mental, or spiritual, is recognized and takes hold at a cellular level. Every lifestyle improvement works toward creating greater and greater health.

It is never too late for a new beginning. That new beginning can be expanded to a greater wholeness by learning how to integrate all three aspects of your Being—body, mind, and spirit.

The Acid/Alkaline Connection:

The body works to maintain within certain ranges the *pH level* of all body fluids and tissue. The pH level is a measure of the balance of acidity and alkalinity. The ideal range of pH varies according to which fluid or tissue is being measured, whether it is blood, stomach, the entire gastrointestinal tract, lymphatic fluids, skin or other tissue.

One of the many problems with the typical American diet is that it can generate too much acid. Examples of high *acid-forming* foods and substances are coffee, tea, sodas, cocoa, alcohol, enriched flour-based foods, sugar, vinegar, catsup, mustard, pepper, cornstarch, tobacco, aspirin and most drugs. Crash dieting and fasting can also upset the acid/alkaline balance because they generate acidic *ketone* bodies.

Some symptoms of *hyper-acidity* might be heartburn and indigestion, burning sensation in the anus, burning urine, halitosis, burning in the mouth and around the tongue, sensitivity to acid fruits or vinegar, bumps on the tongue or roof of the mouth, skin that turns black from jewelry and the inability of the skin to tolerate cosmetics.

On the other hand, *hyper-alkalinity* can occur as well. This could come from eating an overabundance of alkaline-producing food such as fruit and juices. If you are consuming high levels of fruit and may be *juicing*, you are upsetting your acid/alkaline balance. One glass of juice may represent dozens of different fruits in one serving.

Fruit is extremely high in sugar — basically it consists of sugar and distilled water. For example, a glass of orange juice might contain the sugar from ten or more oranges. A large glass of carrot juice could take an entire bag of carrots. That is too much of a sugar surge for the body to handle. When you consume fruit juice, pour out one or two ounces and blend it with pure water or mineral water to dilute the content.

One way to avoid acid/alkaline imbalance is to avoid *mono-meals*. Mono-meals consist of only one or two foods at a meal. A *balanced meal* is made up of foods from all three food groups: protein, carbohydrate and fat. Vegetables, especially raw, always provide a balancing acid/alkaline effect and should be eaten with every meal. Add a raw food because they are easiest to assimilate, richest in nutrients, and are the best source of proper acid/alkaline balance in body fluids and tissue.

The key to maintaining a proper acid/alkaline balance is easy:
At every meal eat a variety of healthy foods, especially
vegetables, from all three food groups.

Your Body -
Judith Speaks!

Δ

After years of working in the area of nutrition and diet, I have observed that people have varying, sometimes startling, relationships with their bodies. These range from no connection to their bodies, to being overly obsessed, to everything in between. Many people are afraid their bodies will somehow undermine or sabotage their existence. Others never take command of their bodies, like a car without a driver, racing out of control.

In fact, many people feel intimidated by their bodies and live their entire existence never daring to learn anything about how it functions. Flying blind, they depend on fate alone to keep them from running into a mountain top.

I find it curious that so many people opt for the *ignorance is bliss* approach to their body and personal health care. Picture yourself taking a hands-off approach to any demanding endeavor such as driving a car, piloting an airplane, or driving a motorcycle with no training. Common sense would compel you to take instructions and master the machine before setting out. Yet, many shun responsibility for the very machine (structure) you are dwelling within. Learning basic principles about how your body functions can make the difference between good and bad health.

Your body is a fantastic machine, possibly the most highly advanced organic system in the universe — certainly the most highly advanced on earth. When people have even a simple understanding of how their bodies function, and are not afraid to climb into the driver's seat, they have a distinct advantage and can improve the quality of their lives. Another way to look at it is that you create harmony when you learn to properly play the instrument. This takes knowledge and practice.

The New Body-Mind-Spirit Approach to Weight Solutions teaches, offers exercises, and demonstrates how to select nutrition and lifestyle options that can help you achieve immediate and long-term goals.

**Most people know how to go on a diet,
yet few know how to continue a weight-loss plan.**

Clients have said to me, "I can lose weight in the first weeks, but I don't know what to do to afterwards." Our Plan offers you an effective start-up and long-term guide for the months and years ahead.

This Plan navigates you through adjustments to diet as well as recommendations for lifestyle changes. It teaches you how to become aware of the three essences of your existence: your body, your mind and your spirit. All three approaches need to integrate in order to make a major impact on your health. We have developed the Plan as a holistic approach to begin your transformation.

Let us move ahead beginning with your physical body.

My Working Journal

A look at my relationship with my body:

<u>Note:</u> Am I like a car without a driver? Do I view my symptoms as a message from my body? Am I in tune with the harmony or dissonance of my body?

_____
_____
_____
_____
_____
_____
_____
_____
_____
_____
_____
_____
_____
_____
_____
_____
_____
_____
_____
_____
_____
_____
_____
_____
_____
_____
_____
_____
_____
_____
_____

Your Body
and Its Biochemistry

Δ

Transforming your Body

It is most encouraging and vastly reassuring to learn that your body has a tremendous regenerative capacity. This rejuvenation force has its genesis deep inside your body at the cellular level where the healing process first begins to work its influence. Over time, the restorative effects emanate outward to the rest of the body.

You may not notice that healing has been initiated by a healthy lifestyle change, and may become discouraged or even give up. You can be unaware for weeks and even months of the changes taking place inside your body. However, they are occurring. Over time, low quality body tissue is broken down and eliminated and newer, healthier body tissue is created in its place.

Stay with a healthy lifestyle program long enough and once unhealthy body systems, such as your digestive system, respiratory system, and endocrine system, begin to function better. You need only improve your nutrition and lifestyle choices for healthy rejuvenation to take place.

The analogy I like to use in describing the pace of healing is if you throw a rock into the middle of a pond, the waves from that impact take their time to reach the shore. Like the shore, you may not initially be aware of the impact, but changes are taking place. Each lifestyle improvement you make and every self-nurturing step you undertake contributes to upgraded cellular activity that brings about greater health.

Your Biochemistry

A body constituent referred to as your *biochemistry* is made up of molecules and compounds including every nutritive compound — vitamin, mineral, antioxidant, bioflavonoid. amino acid, fatty acid, glucose, and so on — that goes into and out of your cells. The high or low *quality* of this biochemical activity against your cells determines your physical health. New research shows that this activity includes:

- *Nutrition* going into our cells.
- Positive or negative *thoughts* impacting our cells.
- Positive or negative *emotions* impacting our cells.
- Positive effect on our cells from *spiritual reflection* and *meditation.*

When you live in a way that positively impacts each of the above, your biochemistry can be transformed from a lower to a higher level of vitality.

As you improve self care in the ways we describe, certain physical characteristics are actually altered. For example, you can change and improve —

- your body's shape and size.
- the tendency of your skin to dry, wrinkle or age.
- the vitality of your hair and nails.
- the strength and durability of joints and bones.
- for women, a tendency toward PMS symptoms.
- for men, prostate symptoms.

> **The experience of poor health today can be transitory and is not necessarily a life sentence.**

According to biochemist, Jeffrey Bland, many of our genetic characteristics are *pleomorphic*, meaning they can express themselves in different ways depending on how they are provoked.

In other words, some genes are fixed and others are changeable. This means that not all of our genetic characteristics are written in stone. This is exciting news because it means that any of us can alter certain aspects of our bodies. You begin by improving your diet. In addition, you become more aware of your lifestyle choices, such as toxic environmental exposures and exposure to damaging chemicals found in your food and water.

> **A transformation of your biochemistry will occur as you consume a healthier diet, supplement with missing nutrients, view yourself in a self-supportive way and spend time in spiritual reflection.**

Altering Your Biochemistry

Many scientists believe that it takes approximately 90 days, on average, to alter the body's biochemistry using natural methods. Measurable physical changes can be observed, even in that short time span. Pharmaceuticals can alter the biochemistry much faster, but the change is contrived and not natural to the body. It takes longer to directly influence the inner workings of our bodies using a natural approach.

It is never too late to transform your biochemistry in a way that improves overall health and wellness. The first step is to make an honest assessment of your current health status. The second step is to increase your knowledge of important health principles. Many people are experiencing poor health today because they never learned basic nutrition and consequently do not understand its impact on their biochemistry.

> **A deficiency in just one single nutrient can have serious consequences.**

Your body is a machine that requires high caliber fuel, in the form of daily nutrients, in order to maximize performance. A deficiency in just one single nutrient can have serious consequences. For example a deficiency of Thiamin can affect our energy levels. A Vitamin B-12 deficiency can cause serious neurological symptoms. A Zinc deficiency can result in lowered immune system function.

Taking Responsibility

Optimum health is not an entitlement but a personal responsibility. As you increase your knowledge of basic nutrition and mind-spirit balance, you are on the path toward integration. By taking control of, rather than abdicating, your personal health care, you achieve body, mind, and spirit fulfillment.

Our goal is to help you recognize that the present level of your health will determine how well, or how poorly, you feel each day. There is no need for physical degradation to begin in mid-life. The ailments that greet you now may be the consequence of prior neglect, but they can also be viewed as a wake-up call. You may feel tired and run down, or suffer from a range of symptoms. If so, it would be beneficial to evaluate your history of dietary and lifestyle choices thus far in tandem with a commitment to change. You have the power to improve the way you feel.

**It is never too late to transform your physical health.
We are never so perfect that we cannot benefit from
improvements in personal caretaking and lifestyle choices.**

Practical applications of transformation begin with a new, and improved, look at fats in our diet.

My Working Journal

What I am learning about my own biochemistry:

<u>Note:</u> What is the quality of the nutrition going into my cells? What steps can I take that directly affect the nutrition going into my cells? What thoughts are affecting my cells? What steps can I take that directly affect the thoughts and emotions impacting my cells?

_____
_____
_____
_____
_____
_____
_____
_____
_____
_____
_____
_____
_____
_____
_____
_____
_____
_____
_____
_____
_____
_____
_____
_____
_____
_____
_____

Your Body
and Low-Fat Diets

Δ

During the last several decades, many Americans began restricting fats due to a theory called the *lipid hypothesis*, which links saturated fat to coronary heart disease (CHD). But before *you* jump to the same conclusion, let's take a look at whether or not the lipid hypothesis has any validity.

Statistics indicate that deaths from CHD have grown from approximately 8% to 45% of all deaths since the turn of the century. In making the case that the risk of dying from coronary heart disease is increased from eating saturated fat, you should expect there to be solid evidence pointing to an increase in the consumption of saturated fat. Well, surprisingly quite the opposite is true.

It is a fact that during the last century, the more we have reduced our intake of saturated fat, the higher the death rate from CHD has grown. An important question to then ask is if we are eliminating the alleged cause, why has the CHD death rate increased?

Another weakness in the argument supporting the lipid hypothesis relates to our massive consumption of low-fat and no-fat foods. These diets are now the norm and one would expect coronary heart disease to decrease as a result. However, CHD disease rates continue to increase year after year. Medical intervention (e.g., bypass surgery and angioplasty) may have had an effect in reducing the death rate somewhat, but lowered fat intake has not. An argument can actually be made that death from coronary heart disease may have *increased* as a result of *fat deficiencies* in the human diet.

How can the long-held belief in the lipid hypothesis be rationalized? Common sense alone dictates that if saturated fat intake was the culprit, CHD death rates would quite naturally decrease with a reduction in consumption. Before you eliminate or restrict fats due to blind faith in the lipid hypothesis, consider these facts:

Before 1920, coronary heart disease was rare. Yet —
- butter consumption was 18 lbs. per person per year.
- eggs, cream and cheese were eaten daily.
- the typical diet averaged 30 grams per day of fat from animal sources.

Since 1920, coronary heart disease has risen exponentially to become responsible for nearly half of all deaths in the United States. Yet —
- butter consumption has decreased from 18 lbs. to 4 lbs. per person per year.
- people are avoiding eggs and cream, and are consuming low-fat dairy products.
- since 1975, the typical daily diet has averaged less than 10 grams of fat from animal sources.
- consumption of refined sugars and starches has increased by 60%.
- consumption of margarine, shortening, and other fake fats has increased by 400%.

(Information from *Nourishing Traditions*, by Sally Fallon and Mary Enig, Ph.D.)

The *Framingham Heart Study* is often quoted as supporting the lipid hypothesis. But, in fact, this 40-year study of approximately 6,000 people failed to prove that theory. According to renowned lipid biochemist, Dr. Mary Enig:

> Investigators claimed that there was a 240% increase in "risk" of coronary heart disease in those having cholesterol levels between 182 and 244. But the actual rate of increase was only .13%. For those with cholesterol levels between 244 and 294, the rate of CHD actually declined. Thus, Framingham investigators found virtually no difference in heart disease for serum cholesterol levels between 182 and 294 — the vast majority of the U.S. population. (Diet and Heart Disease: *Not What You Think. Consumers Research Magazine*, July 1996.)

The *Framingham Heart Study* is not the only research that has failed to prove the lipid hypothesis. Other studies, such as the *Multiple Risk Factor Intervention Trial* (MRFIT) of 362,000 men, showed only a tiny (.1%) increased risk in annual heart disease deaths when comparing cholesterol levels of 180 to levels of 300. This study actually showed *more* of an increase in total deaths when cholesterol levels were below 160. *Low* cholesterol levels are worrisome because they can create a severe hormonal imbalance and other serious health complications.

The *Lipid Research Clinics Coronary Primary Prevention Trial* (LRC), a very expensive study funded by the National Institutes of Health (NIH), compared two groups. One group received a cholesterol lowering drug, and the other a placebo. Independent researchers who later recalculated the published outcome data could find no difference in CHD death rates between the two groups tested. But, a more frightening discovery never publicized was the increase in deaths due to violence and suicide within the drug-taking group.

Danish scientist, Dr. Ufe Ravnskov, has spent more than 20 years reviewing the scientific methods used in developing the lipid hypothesis. As a result, he declared *the diet-heart idea as hopelessly incorrect.* Dr. Ravsnkov, who wrote *The Cholesterol Myths*, is only one of a growing number of eminent researchers that may have been alienated from the medical community due to his dissenting view. But as well known lipid biochemist Michael Gurr states, "By contrast, many who support the consensus view have made their reputations in this field...and have a vested interest in continuing to support and sustain...the idea."

There are enough study results and retrospectives that cast suspicion on the lipid hypothesis. Anyone who takes the time to look at the data will be amazed that the theory has managed to gain support for so long. Yet even while more doctors and researchers are convincingly counter-positioning the lipid theory, the general public remains in the dark and resolute. We find that even with good cause most people are fearful — even terrified — of adding fat back into their diets due to a concern of compromising their cardiovascular health. Convincing people of the importance of putting fat back into their diet has become a colossal challenge to many of us in the health profession.

If not saturated fats, then what other cause or causes of coronary heart disease are lurking in the shadows? There are actually many theories that attempt to answer that question, but let's take a cursory look at two major suspects and the flood into the marketplace of fabricated, highly processed foods such as:

- refined sugars and starches (enriched and fortified food products).
- hydrogenated and other highly processed *plastic* fats and oils.

Refined sugars and starches can be linked to heart disease for two reasons. One, the body converts excess carbohydrates into fat, including stored fat and cholesterol. Two, the over consumption of refined, enriched carbohydrates makes us fatter and can increase cholesterol levels to alarming proportions. A massive health challenge, including higher levels of heart disease and diabetes, has resulted from our subsisting on these overly processed *convenience* foods.

As an example, have you read the sugar labels on typical low-fat foods? They can be as high as 60 grams of carbohydrates per serving. When you multiply 60 grams by four (1 gram of carbohydrates = 4 calories) to ascertain the total number of calories you are consuming, a single serving can reach a total of 240 calories from carbohydrates alone.

Processed carbohydrates seem to dominate the American diet. But, it's no wonder; the food pyramid recommends 6–11 servings per day. Have you actually tried to envision yourself carrying out that suggestion? It means you would have to eat at least two to four servings of bread and cereal-type food with every meal! It is no small wonder that Americans are overweight!

These foods are typically described on labels as containing "enriched flour" and include breads, rolls, muffins, bagels, croissants, scones, pizza, cookies, cakes, cold cereal, pasta, and so on, which many people practically live on.

Refined, enriched flour foods are what nutritionists call fast-acting carbohydrates; this means they surge the bloodstream with glucose. This is largely because the fiber has been removed. Without the fiber to slow its release into the blood stream, the blood sugar surges.

Processed sugars and enriched flour products are really disguised fat calories ratcheting up the pounds on our scales, even though the product packaging may say "No Fat" or "Low Fat."

The consumption of hydrogenated oils such as margarine, shortening and other *fake fats* like olestra and Olean, are causing serious harm to our bodies. It seems more than coincidental that as consumption of these highly altered fats and oils has risen, and the consumption of unprocessed plant and animal fats has decreased, the incidence of coronary heart disease increased. Evidence shows that an appropriate amount of naturally derived saturated fat offers a protective mechanism to all aspects of function in the body.

In the book, *Nourishing Traditions*, Sally Fallon and Dr. Mary Enig describe how vegetable oils and hydrogenated oils are typically processed in the United States:

The oil extraction process:
- Oils are processed in large factories.
- Seeds or nuts are crushed and heated to 230 degrees.
- Oil is squeezed out at 10 to 20 tons per inch, generating more heat.
- Solvents, such as gasoline, hexane, benzene, ethyl ether, and carbon tetrachloride are used in the extraction process.
- The process creates high temperatures, destroying nutrients.
- Natural preservative Vitamin E is lost due to extreme heat.
- Synthetic preservatives, such as BHA and BHT, are added to replace destroyed Vitamin E.
- Overall processing damages fat molecules in a way that is harmful to the body.
- Free radicals, which are unstable particles, are created. These are known to cause cellular and tissue damage inside our arteries.

These are the fats and oils used in most packaged and processed foods. They also represent the typical bottles of oil on our grocery store shelves.

As if this were not bad enough, the oils are further processed to lengthen their shelf life. A typical box of processed food may have a one year shelf life, but using hydrogenated oils lengthens the shelf life many years.

The hydrogenation process (e.g., margarine, shortening, trans-fats, olestra, Olean):
- Manufacturers begin with oils from the extraction process. (Remember, these are already damaged and rancid materials.)

- Oils are mixed with tiny metal particles — usually nickel oxide (very toxic and impossible to totally remove from the end product).
- Soap-like emulsifiers are squeezed into the mixture for consistency.
- Oil is again heated to high temperatures when steam cleaned to remove the horrible odor from emulsifiers and metals.
- Bleaches are often used to improve the unappealing gray coloration.
- Cold tar dyes and strong flavors are added to margarine to make it resemble butter.
- Mixtures are compressed and packaged, ready to be used in your kitchen.

Hydrogenated oils, also called trans-fats, are dangerous because they have become toxic and damaging substances. Their over consumption is being linked to illness and disease.

Hydrogenated oils block the use of Essential Fatty Acids, which have extremely important functions in the body. Essential Fatty Acids —
- keep saturated fats mobile in the blood stream.
- keep cell membrane strong.
- prevent blood cell clumping.
- transport oxygen from red blood cells to tissue.
- enhance nerve transmission.
- balance cholesterol levels.
- minimize inflammation.
- strengthen immune system response.

To avoid these unhealthy oils, shop for cold-pressed oils, such as olive oil and cold-pressed sesame seed oil, and always select butter over margarine or shortening. To be safe, when you are dining out always ask for olive oil on salads.

Similar to Rachel Carson, who warned us in *Silent Spring* of the dangers to the outer environment, the work of Dr. Enig and others may be an important wake-up call warning us of the severe dangers to our inner environment. In fact, we are beginning to see more references in the literature to the dangers of hydrogenated oils. Yet the food industry continues to market and sell margarine, shortening and fake butter spreads as healthy foods. They also continue to use hydrogenated or partially hydrogenated oils in snack and convenience food. It would benefit us to pay attention to Dr. Enig's caution that our *best defense is to avoid trans-fats like the plague.*

> **If we haven't totally lost you to the depth of despair, we have good news. You only need to stop consuming these products in order for your body to begin eliminating them.**

So then, which fats and oils *are* safe for us to consume? In order to optimize the health of our cardiovascular and other systems, it would be wise to select from those indicated below:

> **Choose daily from these healthy fat sources:**
> - Fish and fish oils, such as cod liver oil
> - Organically produced dairy products
> - Hormone and other additive-free poultry and beef
> - Nuts, seeds and unprocessed nut and seed butters
> - Avocado, olives, leafy greens, sea vegetables

> **For cooking**
> - Butter
> - Virgin olive oil
> - Cold-pressed sesame seed oil

> **On salads or hot veggies**
> - Virgin olive oil
> - Walnut or almond oil
> - Flaxseed oil

Now that you have a clearer understanding of the need for naturally derived fats in your diet, let's explore how low-fat diets can result in carbohydrate cravings. As mentioned, it is interesting that Americans have been eating low-fat diets for weight loss for more than 30 years and yet obesity has steadily increased. This is a clear example of being lost in the weight-loss maze.

My Working Journal

What I'm learning about low-fat diets:

_____

_____

_____

_____

_____

_____

_____

_____

_____

_____

_____

_____

_____

_____

_____

_____

_____

_____

_____

_____

_____

_____

_____

_____

_____

_____

_____

_____

_____

_____

_____

_____

Note: Have I been avoiding fats due to the fat myth media hype? How can I shift to a new pattern using healthy fats? When do I start?

Your Body and Carbohydrate Cravings

Δ

I have written an entire section on carbohydrates because I believe it is the most misunderstood and most abused of all the food groups. In order to achieve your desired weight-loss goals, it helps to understand how carbohydrates work in your body and how you can manage them effectively.

Most people believe that weight gain occurs when more calories are consumed than are burned in any given day. While this principle is true, it is only true in part. We can actually gain weight after every meal and every snack in any given day! In other words, we can be putting on weight three to five times a day, if we are eating *glycemic* (blood sugar raising) meals or snacks.

I have seen in my practice that when clients learn how to *glycemically-balance* their carbohydrate intake at every meal and every snack, they can manage weight levels more effectively, especially over the long term.

What is a Carbohydrate?

As a general rule of thumb, carbohydrates are referred to as *sugars and starches*. The body utilizes these sugars as its primary energy source. This *potential energy* develops inside the plant through the action of the sun. This process is *photosynthesis*. Sugars are stored inside plants, like little battery cells, ready to be eaten and converted to glucose, the primary energy source for the body. Once converted, glucose moves into the bloodstream (blood sugar) and is available as a quick source of energy for the body's intellectual and physiological demands.

It helps to differentiate carbohydrates from the other two food groups as any food that *grows*, that is to say most any plant food, with a couple of exceptions. Some exceptions are nuts, seeds, avocados and olives. These also grow as plants, but are higher in fat than in sugar. Nevertheless, most green plant foods — grains, beans, legumes, vegetables, fruits, vegetable and fruit derivatives, all flour, breads, rolls, pasta, muffins, bagels, croissants, desserts, other baked goods, cereals, and juices — are high in carbohydrates.

Carbohydrates are the foods we depend upon for energy, especially quick energy, but are enormously over-consumed by most people.

It is critically important for you to understand carbohydrates (sugars) as a food group if you wish to lose weight and maintain weight levels. That is because continuing to live on fast-acting glycemic carbohydrates makes it difficult, if not impossible, to succeed.

Fast-acting (glycemic) and Slow-acting (less glycemic) Carbohydrates

What makes a carbohydrate a glycemic or less glycemic sugar? In a word: *fiber*. All carbohydrates come to us from Mother Nature containing varying levels of fiber. Low-fiber carbohydrates are more glycemic, and high-fiber carbohydrates are less glycemic.

Glycemic sugars = weight gain
Lower or non-glycemic sugars = weight management

Fiber is the part of the plant that is referred to as cellulose. Some fiber is indigestible and passes intact through your GI tract providing bulk and cleansing toxins. Fiber also inhibits or slows down the absorption of sugar into your blood stream. Foods high in fiber release their sugars from your small intestines into your bloodstream slowly, like a time-released capsule, throughout the morning or the afternoon, as you need the energy.

Alternatively, low-fiber and no-fiber foods can release their sugars into your bloodstream fast and all at once, creating a high blood sugar situation. The body opposes high blood sugar and responds by producing insulin that works to remove the excess. Unfortunately, for most adults and many children, the excess has to go somewhere and is stored inside fat cells.

You can avoid weight gain by glycemically balancing every meal and every snack.

There are three ways to glycemically balance meals. Always include a:
1: high fiber food serving
2: fat or oil serving
3: protein serving

Pay attention to meal planning in a way that balances your carbohydrate serving with at least two of the three choices above. Of course your carbohydrate should ideally be a low-glycemic choice, like brown rice. If it is not, you will need to balance that higher glycemic serving with *all three* of the above choices.

For example, a baked potato (higher glycemic) should be balanced with a protein serving (fish or chicken) and large salad (fiber) with a serving of feta cheese with 1 Tbs. of olive oil (fat) on the salad.

The most highly consumed glycemic, and therefore fattening, food in our country is *enriched, wheat-flour*. Read labels. You will see it makes up much of the American diet and is the reason, I believe, we are the most overweight nation in the world. Take an honest look at your diet. If you are depending on these foods as your primary nutrition, you will never consistently lose weight, or maintain your hard earned weight loss — until you learn to avoid these foods and balance all carbohydrates in the way we have described.

Avoid also refined sugars and sweeteners. The refining process removes the fiber and all important nutrients that originated in the plant from Mother Nature. The fiber and nutrients present in the *whole,* unrefined sweetener are there for a reason. They are necessary to aid in the digestion and metabolism of these sugars. Imbalances can occur when they are not present.

Don't eat these fast-acting sugars:
▲ enriched, wheat flour foods
▲ pre-packaged convenience foods
▲ refined sugar: white table sugar, brown sugar, corn syrup,
    high fructose corn syrup, malto-dextrin
▲ anything ending in *ose:* sucrose, fructose, glucose, dextrose,
    maltose, carbohydratose

Do:
▲ choose natural sweeteners in small amounts (1 tsp. or less):
    ▪ raw honey, real maple syrup, blackstrap molasses
    ▪ dehydrated cane sugar (Sucanat)
    ▪ fresh or frozen fruit
▲ always balance starchy vegetables and fruit with:
    ▪ protein serving
    ▪ healthy fat serving
    ▪ high-fiber food serving

Traditional societies and health conscious individuals who have low levels of heart disease prefer natural sweeteners in moderation.

> **Natural sweeteners are high in vitamins, minerals and fiber**
> **that are not stripped away as they are in the refined versions.**

My Working Journal

My issues with carbohydrates:

Note: Do I over eat carbohydrates? How can I switch from fast- to slower-acting carbohydrates? Am I consuming enough fiber in my daily diet?

_____

_____

_____

_____

_____

_____

_____

_____

_____

_____

_____

_____

_____

_____

_____

_____

_____

_____

_____

_____

_____

_____

_____

_____

_____

_____

_____

_____

_____

Easy Reference for Blood Sugar (Glycemic) Control

Fast-Acting Sugars (Glycemic Carbohydrates)

Eliminate or avoid these foods as they are empty of fiber and low in essential nutrients and can provoke or trigger cravings. It pays to read labels carefully.

▲ **White, enriched flour products:** breads, rolls, muffins, scones, croissants, bagels, pizza, pretzels, enriched flour macaroni, pastas, noodles, pancakes, cookies, cakes, pies, and all desserts or breakfast foods made with enriched flour.

▲ **White rice and instant foods:** white rice, instant oatmeal, instant potatoes, rice cakes, any other puffed instant starch or instant grain food, and dry commercial cereals of all kinds. (The one exception that we have found that can be eaten occasionally is *Uncle Sam's Cereal*).

▲ **Fruit juice:** It is better to eat the whole fruit rather than the juice, which is concentrated sugar. If you do consume juice, select low glycemic juices like tomato or vegetable juices. Carrot juice is very glycemic — like eating a candy bar.

▲ **Fruits:** Best eaten with balancing foods such as a protein or natural fat serving.

▲ **High-starch vegetables:** corn, white potatoes, beets, and carrots. These should always be balanced with protein, healthy fat and high fiber foods.

▲ **Other glycemic foods to avoid:** millet, orzo, couscous, tapioca, and potato flour. (Bean flours and nut meals are glycemically balanced).

Complex, Slower-Acting Sugars
(Less Glycemic Carbohydrates)

Vegetables:
▲ Leafy greens, tomatoes, artichoke, cabbage family, eggplant, cucumbers, celery, cauliflower, onion, garlic, radishes, rutabaga, snow peas, string beans, snap peas, pea pods, asparagus, water chestnuts, summer squash, zucchini, mushrooms, kohlrabi, leeks, sea vegetables (wakame, hijiki, kelp, nori, etc.).

Whole grains: soaking grains overnight before cooking can be a digestive aid
▲ Cooked grain cereals: oatmeal, cream of rice, cream of wheat, and cream of kasha
▲ Other whole grains such as brown rice, brown basmati rice, and wild rice
▲ 100% whole wheat bulgur, whole wheat couscous, spelt, amaranth, teff
▲ 100% whole rye, buckwheat, kamut, quinoa

Breads:
▲ Sprouted-grain bread products such as Ezekiel or whole-grain sour dough bread

Beans: beans contain the highest fiber levels of all plant foods
▲ Whole bean foods, such as adzuki, black, garbanzo, kidney, lentils, lima, soybeans, pinto, navy, white, red, yellow, whole pea beans, etc., and hummus and other bean spreads

Nuts and seeds: also high in fiber
▲ Almonds, cashews, filberts, hazelnuts, pecans, pine nuts, walnuts, macadamia nuts, pumpkin seeds, sesame seeds, sunflower seeds, flax seeds, and natural nut butters

---

Glycemically balance every meal and snack with at least two of the following:
1: one high fiber food serving
2: one healthy fat or oil serving
3: one protein serving

My Working Journal

The list of glycemic foods that I consume daily:

_____
_____
_____
_____
_____
_____
_____
_____
_____
_____
_____
_____
_____
_____
_____
_____
_____
_____
_____
_____
_____
_____
_____
_____
_____
_____
_____
_____
_____
_____
_____
_____
_____
_____
_____

Note: Which glycemic foods do I crave? Do I eat glycemic foods by
themselves (e.g., dry cereals, bread, bagels, desserts, or fruit)?

Your Mind –
Janet Speaks!
Δ

If you have excess body fat that you cannot lose...
If you have dieted and lost weight only to regain it...
If self-help tapes and books haven't worked for you...
If you keep repeating the same unproductive patterns...
If you are feeling negative about your lack of success...
Stop. Take time out to seek your underlying motives!
There are reasons!

There is a reason for all things — and those reasons are often locked in your unconscious mind. You are a product of all of your thoughts, programming, beliefs, and experiences. Your unconscious mind is the Powerhouse...and it will work for or against your conscious goals.

It is my strong belief, based upon personal and professional experiences, that we must *balance* our energies among our mental, emotional, physical and spiritual *selves* for optimum health. I have seen so many clients who are focused on their physical bodies while their *spirits are starving* for fulfillment. That sense of hunger is interpreted as physical hunger. Often, one tries to fill the emptiness with food. It will not work.

Physical hunger must be filled physically.
Emotional hunger must be filled emotionally.
Mental hunger must be filled mentally.
Spiritual hunger must be filled spiritually.

I am a counselor and specialist in regression therapy — taking a person back into memory. Regression therapy can help a person find the *root cause* of self-defeating patterns. By locating the blockage and releasing stored emotion, there is a release of energy from the unconscious mind to conscious awareness. You are then free to begin to create new habit patterns. As long as the blockage remains, it is very difficult to move ahead to success and happiness. The memories or decisions in the unconscious mind hold you back.

I constantly encourage you to listen to yourself. It is in this way that you begin to get in touch with that lost or buried part of you — a part that you may have concealed in excess body fat. How have you done that?

- By blocking your energy.
- By stuffing down your emotions.
- By keeping your own personality and inner being hidden.
- By negating and/or devaluing your intuition and sensitivity.
- By your lack of self-expression.

In other words...by losing touch with who you are!

You Are Your Own Expert!

You have been taught to go to the experts. Diet and exercise gurus abound, with

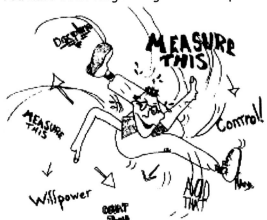

little impact for the person with a chronic weight problem. It is time to *stop* looking outside of yourself for the answers. No one knows you better than you know yourself, and if you have been ignoring your*self* — more correctly your*selves* — this workbook can help to change that.

My work in obesity and weight control now spans more than 35 years as I moved from teaching diet, nutrition, behavior modification and exercise, to reprogramming the mind through visualization and hypnosis, to seeking the *cause* through regression therapy.

Over the past three decades, there has been so much information about losing weight that *every person who is overweight knows how to lose weight*. Why then have the statistics not improved? Today obesity has sky rocketed among children as well as adults. In spite of an increased interest in fitness and health, statistics report the same shocking reality; more than 90% of dieters who lose weight gain it back.

We have focused in the wrong direction. Many so-called experts[1] continue to emphasize externals (diet change, exercise, behavior) and avoid internal factors (thoughts, beliefs, mind patterning, and emotions). Clearly we have not addressed the mind's ability to hold unconscious reasons to keep excess body fat. Nor have we begun to consider the spirit or energy essence of the individual. *Experts* continue to study the effect instead of the cause.

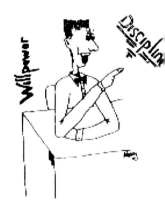

Good nutrition and exercise are, of course, necessary for a healthy, normal body weight. Yet, there are millions of obese and/or overweight people who cannot — *cannot* —lose weight and keep it off.

**Less-than understanding friends and some experts cry out, "You just need more willpower." Willpower is a function of the conscious mind.
Can you lose weight with willpower? Of course. It happens
all the time...and any diet or exercise program will work for a time.
If, however, there are *reasons* held in your unconscious mind to keep the excess fat, you will gain all the weight back.**

Do I make it sound like a battle? It is. If you have lost weight and gained it back again and again, you know that it is a horrendous battle. It is an *internal* fight, a fight between the conscious mind that says, "I really want to lose weight" and the unconscious mind that says, "I need the weight because...". Obesity is an

---

[1] The only "expert" on you is *you!* We trust that you will listen to yourself for your answers.

internal fight. And, any *external* measures, although valuable, cannot solve the problem alone.

> **The problem is not the cause.**
> **The cause is internal — the cause is in the mind.**

Those internal causes are the experiences of the person that have brought about a *need* for extra layers of body fat for protection. The cause is locked in your unconscious mind.

One of the most discouraging facts of the weight-loss battle is that the dieter loses hope. Each new effort is fueled with the underlying belief (and fear) that you will just gain it all back. When you recognize that there are reasons why you have put the weight on, you can also understand *that what the mind creates, can be re-created.*

Working in the field of traditional weight-control counseling for several years and seeing this frustrating reality was what led me to move into a deeper study of the mind and hypnosis. I eventually opened my own practice and began working with clients to change habits and re-program the mind to a healthier body image.

Although the success rate improved slightly, I quickly realized that for most life-long dieters, the unconscious mind held memory and programming that was not easily changed. In spite of what I said, many people were still seeking a fast, no-effort answer to losing weight; they wanted me to *hypnotize away their fat.* Others were ready to take responsibility and understood what I was teaching. Yet, I began to understand that for most overweight people, the unconscious mind held programming and beliefs that were not modified by standard hypnosis techniques. For many years now, I have done intensive work related to the deep unconscious mind.

> **Through my education and experience, I learned about the power of the**
> **mind. Through my clients, I learned about the vulnerability of the mind.**

I began doing regressions — taking people back into their childhood memories and experiences — to find the cause of their weight problem.

Your Unconscious Mind

Δ

The blockages in your unconscious mind have prevented you from being free — as surely as if your hands were tied with ropes.

I want to emphasize the difference between your conscious mind and your unconscious mind. Your conscious mind might say, "*I really need to lose weight. I don't feel attractive, my clothes don't fit any more, I huff and puff when I climb stairs, and I don't have any energy.*" You might even gather your willpower to begin a diet and/or exercise program.

> **If your unconscious mind holds *reasons* to keep the excess body fat, you will either sabotage yourself, or successfully lose the weight only to gain it all back.**

Through my work in regression therapy, I learned that many people have a *need* to keep excess body fat. That need for fat is a need for protection, in response to memories locked in their unconscious minds.

What memories would trigger your need to keep excess body fat? Of course such memories are unique to each person's life and experiences. They may include:
- Food programming: early training in what to eat, how to eat, when to eat, and why one eats.

- Childhood experiences of early parenting — being overly-disciplined, smothered with over attention, or being ignored — and the child's emotional and mental responses to such experiences.
- Shame about one's body due to messages from family members and classmates at school (e.g., the teasing and embarrassment).
- Physical, emotional, mental, and, for some, sexual abuse.

Some of these issues or memories could be discussed during counseling sessions, and often are. There is quite a difference, however, when an adult discusses a memory with the rational mind, and when that same adult *relives* the experience in hypnosis. Even though the client is completely aware of talking to me and is conscious of the surroundings, early childhood emotions as a child are often remembered and felt.

The mind stores not only the event, but also the feelings and emotions connected with that event. *Feeling memories* are stored at the time that they happened. Clients have been surprised at the emotions they feel when reliving an experience in hypnosis. A memory that can be talked about in a rational, adult manner, takes on a completely different tone when the client relives it as a five year old child.

> **We are truly a product of all of our thoughts, memories, beliefs, and experiences. First comes thought — then comes the physical manifestation of that thought. Your thoughts are a major factor in creating your reality, which is the prism through which you see the world.**

When I speak of the mind, I am not talking about brain or the intellect. When I speak of mind, I refer to consciousness — and consciousness is held within every cell of your body and is also the energy that moves out from your physical body. Consciousness *includes* your emotional, mental, and spiritual selves, an energy flow encompassing the whole — your *greater mind*.

Your conscious mind is the more rational, logical, physically-alert part. It has the ability to do deductive reasoning and is more connected to your ego and the personality that you project.

> **Your unconscious mind is the storehouse of everything that has happened to you since your birth — and research in consciousness indicates even before birth — until the present time.**

It is very important for you to understand more about your unconscious mind. For example, any event that you witnessed, anything important that another person said or did to you, and any situation that you experienced is held within your unconscious mind, and can be replayed at any time. These memories can be replayed at a conscious level, as you remember what happened last week or when you were a teenager. They can also be replayed at an unconscious level. This is when something moves through your mind and you are not aware that it has occurred. All of those subtle movements of memory and feeling continue to affect us on a daily basis.

Your unconscious mind contains not only memory, but also the *feelings and emotions connected with that memory*. I have found in my work with clients in hypnosis that stored feelings and emotions attached to memory contribute to their lack of success. Between birth and approximately age six, your unconscious mind was very open and receptive. Most of what you heard and perceived was taken in *as fact*. Your unconscious mind absorbs, yet does not have the ability to do deductive reasoning.

> **Thought is energy. Emotion is energy. Fat is energy.**
> **Excess fat means that energy is not moving or flowing freely throughout the body-mind system. Excess fat is blocked energy.**

As we feel the need to protect ourselves, we put on excess layers of fat. And there are very good reasons to keep layers of fat for protection...as far as the unconscious mind is concerned.

Excess body fat is *one form* of manifesting blocked energy. I don't want anyone to get the impression that I am saying thin people have no blockages. They simply manifest those (sometimes same or similar) blockages in other ways. I am talking about energy and energy can take a variety of pathways. For example, energy blocks can create or contribute to emotional or mental imbalances, as well. If you are a human being, you do have energy blockages.

Fat serves as a protective layer. There are many individual reasons why a person has an unconscious need to protect the self. I have found five major reasons for manifesting excess body fat.

1. To keep feelings and emotions in.

In my experience, most overweight or obese people are very attuned to their Emotional Self. You may recognize that you feel your emotions strongly. In our society this is not valued. Your sensitive nature doesn't quite fit into our *"don't act emotional, be cool"* western society. And so you try to adapt. To adapt requires a *shutting down*, closing down your sensitivity, blocking your Emotional Self. The body responds to that *need* at an unconscious level. Layers and layers of body fat *will dull* your receptive, Emotional Self.

You might learn that you eat to *stuff the emotions down* to avoid feeling your emotions as they begin to rise. To keep them in — to avoid their expression — food is abused. And it works! Eating *will* stuff it and keep emotions in.

▲ In therapy, Cynthia discussed her teen years when her friends started to date. Cynthia's pleasant personality was an asset to friendship with boys, but no one invited her out on a date. She sat on her bed, reading teen magazines and munching on chips, sipping sodas, and crunching cookies as she pretended that she *didn't want to go to the prom anyway.*

▲ Marie is a lovely hostess. Family members and their children, as well as friends, drop in unannounced because Marie can always handle it. The smile that Marie has *pasted* on her face, however, denies her honest reaction. "It's not fair," she said to me, "they expect me to feed them, pick up after them, do extra laundry, and they're flitting off to visit friends." Does she tell them? No, she eats more leftovers.

▲ Henrietta has been obese all her life. She is a very emotional person. Her husband is an engineer whose nature is to stay in his head, speaking from his logical mind. Displays of outward emotion make him extremely uncomfortable, in fact, quite disgusted, which he voices in no uncertain terms to Henrietta. It becomes a *daily task* (unconsciously) for Henrietta to push her Emotional Self down in order to be the person her husband wants her to be.

2. To keep personal power down.

Power is energy. Energy is power. How comfortable are you with your own power? Do you think in negative or positive terms when you imagine a powerful person? I have found that a majority of overweight clients keep their power down. They prefer to stay passive and, in fact, do not even recognize or have a sense of their own personal power. Do you identify with this? If so, you might recognize that in relationships, you give your power away to avoid risk or change. You fear hurting others' feelings, and are fearful of being hurt. You might accept, give in, give up, and avoid, rather than act in your own behalf. If this is your pattern, examine the reasons and discover where this started for you.

▲ Mildred could not understand why she was not able to stay on a diet. Her doctor insisted that she lose weight, yet every weight-loss program that she tried ended in failure. I moved our discussion away from food to what was happening in Mildred's life. The subject of her grandchildren quickly came up. Mildred loved her grandchildren, but was becoming increasingly frustrated.

She had become an *automatic babysitter* whenever her son and his wife went out. When they needed a vacation, the three grandchildren stayed with Mildred and her husband. Did they check with her schedule or consider finding additional support? No. Did Mildred's husband share the load? No. Did Mildred speak up? No. Rather than expressing her own independence or need for a life of her own, Mildred continued to *give herself away*. She did what everyone else wanted her to do. In order to keep her own power (energy) down, she ate.

▲ Barbara's husband openly disapproved of her excess weight. She had been thin when they were married, but the extra 35 lbs. on her small frame made her feel and look matronly. Barbara tried dieting with failure after failure. She bought ice cream for the family and kept it in the basement freezer. Barbara would sneak downstairs and eat ice cream from the box so her husband would not know. More than once, she threw away empty half-gallon containers that she had spooned through *without his knowledge.* Barbara was unable to stand up for herself as an adult and speak to her husband, saying, "I am going to enjoy a small dish of ice cream." Instead, she viewed him as being *in charge* of her eating behavior. Like a little girl sneaking away from the authority of the father figure, Barbara preferred to act out a powerless position in their relationship.

▲ Sheila holds a high-level position in a successful computer company. She and Howard have been married for 17 years; a second marriage for both of them. Sheila speaks only in the most positive and glowing terms about Howard and their marriage. If a friend asks how Sheila is, she hears how well Howard is doing. Sheila is an attractive, articulate and capable woman. Howard is a hard worker, capable, but insecure. Sheila is constantly giving her energy to boost Howard's self-esteem. When he retired, *fueling his ego* became a full-time job. Sheila automatically puts herself in a lesser position to try to lift the way Howard is perceived in the eyes of others. As long as she suppresses her own power, she continues to gain weight.

3. To avoid stored memories.

There is a desire to avoid the emotion stored in painful memories. Of course, who among us wants to relive the pain of the past? *Let it stay buried. Why dig all that up,* I've heard. I would agree...*if* we were not affected by those memories. The truth of the matter is, all of our past has made us who we are today. And if your memories include being called names as a child, laughed at while playing games at recess, being left out, your greatest healing comes by allowing the memory and acknowledging the pain. Then, you can be free to move forward.

Some memory is even more devastating. Statistics indicate that three out of five women have been sexually abused. I have worked with many such women in hypnosis and I can tell you that sexual abuse affects every level of consciousness. Healing from such traumatic memories takes time.

There is physical abuse, as well as mental and emotional abuse. Often this was directed to us by well-intentioned parents or others who were acting out of their own hurt. If this is your experience, seek out a therapist who works with healing the inner child and begin to free yourself from the pain of the past. I encourage you to examine these memories and begin your inner healing.

▲ Tom's father was domineering. Primary memories in his unconscious mind were of his father saying, "You'll never amount to anything," and "You can't do anything right." Although Tom had held an administrative position in a successful company, he always believed that he *got a lucky break*. Tom's weight gain started when his position was eliminated in the company's downsizing. His father's words were translated into Tom's negative self-talk.

▲ Alice had always had a weight problem, but the past few years it had gotten "completely out of control." At first, Alice couldn't connect to any instance that triggered the additional weight. I asked Alice how long it had been since "a little overweight" had changed to obesity. "About five years ago," she replied.

"What else happened in your life five years ago?" I asked. A shocked expression came on her face. "I put my mother in a nursing home." Alice's memory rushed to the surface. "She didn't want to go, but she needed constant medical attention. My husband had just had a heart attack and my two brothers couldn't have her live with them. My mother said, `I can't believe that you are doing this to me.' I felt so guilty. I never thought I'd ever put a parent into a nursing home." Alice's sobbing continued for a long time. She had never connected the additional 80-lb. weight gain that began five years ago with the internal trauma of the difficult decision she made — five years ago.

4. To punish yourself.

A lack of self love or deep unconscious belief that you deserve to be punished is often uncovered as an obese person begins to take an inner look. Guilt connected to past memories can fuel a desire to punish oneself. A lack of love will contribute to creating a body that cannot be loved and accepted. A belief that you *do not deserve* happiness, a slim attractive body, to speak your opinions, equality in the family structure... equates with self punishment.

▲ Patty lost 75 lbs and looked great. She had been very disciplined with following a diet plan in spite of her husband's inconsiderate attitude. He belittled the food she ate, laughed at marks she put on her calendar for a day of behavior change and exercise, and brought home snacks which he freely ate in front of her. Patty's determination was like steel and her excess fat diminished weekly.

The week she reached her goal, Patty's husband did take notice. She was lovely. He took her on a weekend trip to celebrate — and from that moment on, Patty gradually and consistently gained all the weight back, plus more. I well remember her statement, "I want to show him what he can have, and then show him he can't have it." Patty may think she is punishing her husband; in fact, she is punishing herself.

▲ Minnie remained obese to avoid interacting with men. She believed if she were attractive, men would make passes at her. Like Patty, Minnie was hurting herself.

5. To protect your spirit.

The sensitive person has a need to protect their spirit by hiding it safely away — not letting anyone know the *real you*. Often the spirit has been hurt in early years and the adult is unwilling to be put in such a vulnerable position again.

Sometimes there is a lack of desire to *be here.* There is fear of experiencing life…and a need to avoid the free-flowing energy that exists when one is *fully present and feeling in the body.*

Jovial, clown-like and happy-go-lucky, many obese people use their external personality to cover up their *real* self. Laughing on the outside, crying on the inside may be an exaggeration, but not always. The highly sensitive person will laugh at self before someone else laughs first. It hurts less.

All we need to do is walk through a small group of people, such as in a grocery store, to overhear conversations in which cruel words are spoken to children, or tactless comments are made to family members. When children hear and feel the insensitivity from those who are *supposed to love them,* they are confused and hurt. They begin to *protect* themselves energetically from the onslaught of harmful energy to their spirit.

Watch a young child before he or she has been *conditioned* by adults. The child is free and unashamed about the body; emotions are honest and real; he or she is curious about the environment. As programming continues, depending on its direction and intensity, the child diminishes freedom in order to adapt. Some of the adaptation, of course, is necessary and valuable. Yet much of it is not beneficial. The spirit may become, in time, concealed even from oneself.

I have summarized five of the major reasons for manifesting fat on the body. The *Body-Mind-Spirit Reflections* in this workbook can be used to help you discover your reasons to keep excess weight. To begin, below give a value from 1 to 5 according to your own inner sense of the issue(s) that could be holding you back. Record the number 1 as highest in strength, and 5 as your lowest in strength.

_____To keep feelings and emotions in.
_____To keep personal power down.
_____To avoid stored memories.
_____To punish yourself.
_____To protect your *spirit.*

The Power and Vulnerability
of Your Unconscious Mind

The public is awakening to the power of the mind and the inner connectedness of the mind and body. In fact, there is not a separation — a place where mind *stops* and body *starts*. Occasionally, I have a client say that when they tell friends they are going to a hypnotherapist, comments are, *I'd never do that; no one is going to play around with my mind.* Obviously a credible clinical hypnotherapist does not *play around with* another person's mind. And, do any of us really believe that our mind is *untarnished, unaffected,* or *unblemished* by life? *We have already been programmed!*

We have been programmed by our parents — based upon their programming! We have been programmed by older brothers and sisters, grandparents, and teachers, as well as by our culture, the religious structure we were *born into*, and the society in which we live. The media, and advertising, continue the programming daily. Yes, we *are* vulnerable.

> **Much of our programming includes subtle and not-so-subtle messages that contribute to lowered self-esteem, negative self image, and lowered abilities for success.**

▲ In a discussion about childhood programming, a client told me that in her husband's family, she heard comments about her husband and his sisters all having the "Wilson butt." She was horrified at the comment of her sister-in-law after the birth of her baby. "Look at that, she has the Wilson butt." The newborn infant weighed *six pounds!*

Before we can tap into more of the power of the mind, we need to examine and release some of the garbage. As you examine some of your childhood or teenage messages, you will gain a better understanding of your personal *blockages* to success. "You'll never amount to anything," of course, is an example of a negative message that will continue to affect the child into adulthood.

There will be some things that you will want to keep. I trust that you also have some positive and nurturing messages in your unconscious. "You can be anything you want to be," is an example of a positive message.

You will have opportunities to examine the programming, messages, and suggestions in your unconscious mind. By taking this inner path, you will be able to examine which suggestions are valuable, positive, and productive to you at this time in your life, based on your personal experiences. This will be different from your parents' experiences. In the *Reflections*, you may discover *their* programming which you will want (and need!) to throw out.

> ▲ Martha, a woman in her 70s, came to me because she was disturbed over her weight. Martha's husband was an invalid, bedridden for five years. As a former nurse, she was qualified to care for him, and had adapted to nurturing his constant needs. The few times she left the house for grocery shopping or quick errands, another nurse had to be called. It was obvious that Martha had been under stress for many years.
>
> When I met her, it was near Thanksgiving and she told me that her son and his family would be visiting. I listened in amazement as Martha told me how she had to "get the drapes cleaned, wash the china, and polish the silver." Martha did not realize that she had a choice. She had been raised with programming that certain things were done at certain times. She did not understand that she could make different choices that Thanksgiving.

The *Body-Mind-Spirit Reflections* in this workbook will help you examine your inner messages and programming.

After these discoveries, you can get rid of those inner messages which no longer serve you. Then, you will be ready to create new habit patterns — no longer being sabotaged by the blockages which have unconsciously held you back. Use these reflections as your journal into personal discovery. They are, in fact, your inner journey to learning more about who you are.

By getting in touch with other aspects of yourself, you bring that information into your conscious awareness. It is because it has been locked away, forgotten or hidden, that it has power over you. Release the memory and you diminish that power. Bring it from the cold darkness of your unconscious into the warmth of the light. Examine it — and free yourself.

Your Mental Self

In order to discover your mental blockages, you need to examine your mind at a deeper level. Do you want to lose weight? "Of course I want to lose weight," you scream. "Why do you think I bought this workbook?" Well, that is the *surface stuff*. That is what your conscious mind says. If you have not been successful, if you have lost weight and gained it back again and again, you may have reasons in your *unconscious mind* why you *need* to keep the excess fat.

Consider how often your thoughts dwell upon excess body fat, a closet full of clothes that don't fit, inability or not enough time to exercise, calories, the next meal, sweets or snacking, negative thoughts about your body and the opinion of others about how you look.

> **Be aware that *your internal thoughts affect your external actions.***

If your mind is focused on something, it can bring that about. For example, if your thoughts dwell upon what foods you can't eat on your diet, what you plan to eat at your next meal, how you can avoid overeating at tomorrow's family gathering, or what you'll cook for dinner, you are *concentrating* your attention on food. Through your Mental Self, you are creating a *desire* for food!

> **What you *focus* your attention on, what you give mental energy to, moves you in that direction. Your thoughts — positive or negative — can create addictive behavior.**

The key is: you can control your thoughts, *after* you have cleared your unconscious blockages.

Thoughts can be perceived as internal pictures. Therefore, it is important as you do the *Body-Mind-Spirit Reflections* that you *allow* the inner pictures to automatically arise. This is important because your unconscious mind responds most strongly to internal pictures. By doing this, you will recognize the messages you have been sending to your unconscious mind.

> **You've heard the expression, "What you see is what you get." Your mental picture of yourself can, over time, actually create your external body.**

For years I heard successful dieters say, "Janet, I've lost all this weight, but I still *feel* fat." What they were saying is that their inner image — the way that they continued to *see* themselves — is as a fat person. I can guarantee that every person who said that gained all the weight back!

Research on mind-body interaction has proven that if you cannot *see,* or sense, yourself accomplishing a task, you cannot do it! Your mind must be able to *see* the success — the finished goal, the normal-weight body — in order to bring it about. Consider the current mental image of yourself that you carry in your mind. *Is this the image that you want to create?* Your mind is so powerful; it is essential that you project the healthy, attractive image that you desire in order to bring it into reality.

If you discover, through this workbook, that you have been dwelling upon excess body fat and a negative body image, you *must* change your thought patterns now to effectively change your external image.

Your next step is to examine the messages, both verbal and non-verbal, that you received as a child and continue to receive from the people around you. As much as we would like to deny it, we have been programmed since our birth by the people around us and the society in which we live.

"So," you think, "I have all of these memories and thoughts, but what does it have to do with me today?" Particularly in our younger years, we were learning who we were, our self value, based upon the feedback we got from people around us. At a young age, we began to build a basic belief system about who we were, what we could do, or could not do.

> ▲ As a child, Philip was not allowed to talk back or to express his opinions. It was common for him to hear, "Because I said so, and I don't want to hear another word about it!" Today, when Philip's boss gives him a task to accomplish with instructions on how it is to be done, it is troubling. Philip's style is different than that of his boss, and often he is not comfortable with the direction. He has a different concept on how the task could be handled, but he can't speak up. He continues to respond as he was programmed to do when he was young.

All of your past has programmed you to be the person that you are today. By examining your unconscious mind and looking at your programming — your Mental Self — you can change your automatic patterned response.

I have had several overweight clients bring me photographs of themselves as a child or their formerly thin selves after having just dieted to reach a goal weight. In each case they expressed amazement, "Look Janet, I wasn't fat. Was I? But I thought I was!" Often it was parents or other family members who contributed to the mental programming by words and actions that reinforced a fat body image. When the child's inner belief is that she is fat, as an adult she usually becomes that image.

> ▲ Pat remembered being thin and sickly as a child. She constantly heard persistent messages to eat in order to "look healthy and good." Now overweight, Pat recognizes that she is still eating to make her mother happy, even though she is an adult and her mother is no longer living.

Unless you have already done a lot of work related to disciplining your mind, there is a good chance that your mind lacks focus. Many of my clients are very scattered with their mental energy. Note, when I refer to disciplining the mind, I'm not talking about controlling your thoughts. Your mind needs to be free for the intuitive impulses of the moment. I'm also not talking about deliberate thinking based upon someone else's suggestions. I'm referring to the ability to know what you choose for your life — and moving your mind in that direction.

Do you choose happiness or unhappiness? A ridiculous question? Most people, of course, would say happiness. And yet, those same people will often dwell upon negative situations which bring about constant unhappy thoughts.

> **Your unconscious mind responds to what you tell it. Fill it with unhappy and negative thoughts, and that is exactly what you will have. That is exactly what you are *choosing!***

Do you choose to be slim and healthy, or fat and unhealthy? Listen to your internal talk. What do you dwell upon? What is your Mental Self creating?

Your internal thoughts will affect your external actions. What do your actions indicate about your self-worth? I often use the analogy of owning a beautiful silk shirt or valuable piece of jewelry. We are inclined to care for the shirt by hanging it up and sending it to the cleaners; we put the jewelry in a safe place where it won't be lost or damaged. Contrast that with how you might treat an old dirty pair of sneakers with holes that you wear to garden. You might toss them down the basement stairs because it doesn't really matter.

If you are *not* nurturing yourself, there are unconscious reasons why you have decided you are not as worthwhile as others. Your self-value is created by your Mental Self — your thoughts, beliefs, and programming related to who you are. Are you willing to nurture yourself as well as you nurture others?

After reading this section, what are you discovering about your *need* for excess fat? Keep in mind that the process of reading works with your conscious mind. However, the *need* for layers of fat as protection *does not reside* in your conscious mind; it resides in your unconscious. It is your unconscious mind that accepted the programming *as fact* and continues to hold onto the need until the blocks are removed. Discussing and sharing with your Workbook Support Group can be a great asset in this regard.

The *Body-Mind-Spirit Reflections* will trigger your unconscious mind. It is important to move the conscious mind and the unconscious mind into agreement before success can be achieved. Remember, we are working with the *whole* mind — and the whole self. The energy of your Mental Self moves and flows through all aspects of your being: your emotions, your spirit, and your physical body.

You cannot escape your mind — your unconscious thoughts. They will work for, or against, your conscious goals. As you examine your inner self, keep those messages that benefit your personal growth and release the negative memories that hold you back.

> **Be aware of your thoughts. Awareness is the first step to change. The good news is: What your mind has created can be re-created.**

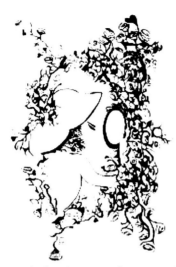

Body-Mind-Spirit Reflections- Phase 1

Δ

Your Body

Reflection 1 ~ Exploring Thoughts and Decisions About Your Body

Let's begin to make some breakthroughs to your Mental Self as it relates to thoughts about your body. We'll do this through some self-evaluation. It is important to write rapidly and spontaneously as thoughts come into your mind. If you wish, use other paper or create a notebook. Allow your mind to be free. You will benefit most by doing this writing the *first time* that you read this section, then adding to your list anytime afterwards.

Throughout this workbook, we will be using your conscious mind and unconscious mind — both sides of your brain. When they are in agreement, instead of fighting each other, you will have an unbeatable combination.

The first step in discovering more about your body perception through your Mental Self is to examine your inner thoughts. Be honest with yourself. Write down your *first* thoughts instead of what you think the "right" answer should be. This is not a test. It is a step toward self-empowerment. You are not seeking anyone else's approval.

Using your *non-dominant hand* (i.e., left hand if you are right-handed), write randomly and rapidly the words that come into your mind.

> [Note: The reason for using your non-dominant hand is that you access a less-used part of your brain. For example, if you are right handed and using

your non-dominant left hand to write, you will be accessing the right hemisphere of your brain, which is considered to be more connected to your unconscious levels of mind].

Describe each part of your body —

Face:

Arms/shoulders:

Chest/breast:

Upper torso:

Waist:

Hips:

Legs:

Feet:

Write words that describe the clothes in your closet:

_____
_____
_____
_____
_____
_____
_____

Write your thoughts about exercise:

_____
_____
_____

Write your thoughts about eating and food:

_____
_____
_____
_____

Reflection 2 ~ Exploring Early Memories Related to Food and Body Messages

Write quickly, allowing your mind to be free. Write down first thoughts; you can expand upon your list later. Think about your childhood and young adulthood.

Remember to use your non-dominant hand in writing.
What messages were you given related to:

Meal time?

_____
_____
_____
_____

Quantities of food?

_____
_____
_____
_____

Types of food?

_____
_____
_____
_____
_____

When to eat?

_____
_____
_____
_____

Reasons you eat?

_____
_____
_____
_____

Now, remember messages received about your size or body shape. What thoughts come to mind? Write them down:

_____
_____
_____
_____

Remember school and classmates. Write down whatever thoughts come to mind. Compare your body size to that of your young friends:

_____
_____
_____
_____
_____

What messages did you receive about your place in the family structure?

_____
_____
_____
_____

Were you encouraged to have private time? Personal space? Your own opinions? Allow yourself to remember how you were treated by each member of the family. Continue to give yourself time. Write down free-floating thoughts:

_____

_____

_____

_____

What are your thoughts when you see an obese person walking down the street?

_____

_____

_____

_____

Write your private thoughts when standing nude before a full-length mirror:

_____

_____

_____

_____

_____

If this applies, what are your inner thoughts about your body when you are with a lover?

_____

_____

_____

_____

_____

Your Emotional Self

Δ

The Connection to Mind

Your feelings and emotions are just as *real* as your fingers and toes. Why then do we so often ignore, dismiss, and deny them? Many of my clients have shut down their feelings and emotions to the point that they are no longer in touch with them. They have lost contact with this greater part of themselves.

Many of us were taught throughout our lives to value and emulate the unemotional figure, male or female, who stands straight, head erect, eyes dry, whether it is at a funeral, a divorce, a wedding, or losing a political race. Some become like robots — cold, unfeeling, masking or covering any honest emotional response. I suggest to you that the stronger figure is one who can freely express his or her Emotional Self, one whose energy is balanced among the body, mind, and emotions.

Many of my overweight clients have strong emotional systems. They are attuned to their emotions, whether they want to be or not. It is a part of who they are. It is a most valuable part of the personality and yet, most of them are stuffing down that part of themselves with food. Food *does* work to dull or drug the emotions; it becomes a way to avoid feeling.

In doing childhood regressions, I often find that these people learned at an early age that their emotions were not allowed. Anger, tears, or even excitement, the child learned that expressing such emotion was frowned upon, and often punished.

What do you *do* with emotion then? You quickly learn to keep it inside, to stuff it down. Hold the tears in, hold the anger in, hold the fear in, and even hold the joy in — because when you stuff down the emotion, you stuff it all. You cannot say to yourself, "I'll keep the anger and fear inside and only feel my excitement and joy and love." No, it cannot be done. Unfortunately, the barriers you put up to your Emotional Self exist to avoid all feeling.

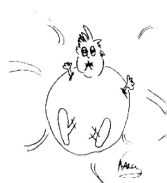

You might say, "That's not me. I cry easily." Do you really let the tears flow or do they quickly rise to the surface where you can dab your eyes and be done with it?

Or, perhaps sadness is an emotion that you can express but anger is out of the question. What emotion are you least capable of exposing?

> ▲ During a counseling session, I referred to a client's anger toward a parent. She looked at me with surprise and calmly said, "Angry? Janet, I'm not angry." It was an honest response; she did not believe that she had any anger. It was nearly a year and a half later when she called me up and said, "I'm so angry, I can hardly stand it!" She had reached the anger that had been stored inside for approximately 35 years.

I have had clients so fearful of showing their emotional side (in their eyes, making fools of themselves) that they medicated themselves out of feeling. Others create a strong shell around themselves. Some become very detached from relationships, from family, and even from themselves. This pattern becomes so much a way of life that the person equates the pattern with the personality — the pattern *becomes* the personality. Understand, I'm talking about energy.

Emotion is energy. Blocked emotion is blocked energy. Blocked energy can manifest in excess fat on the physical body.

As I said, emotions are just as real as any part of your body. Ignoring them or pretending they don't exist does not work any more than you could pretend that you don't have a nose.

> ▲ Sam is a sensitive man who grew up in a family with a domineering father who would not permit any emotional expression, especially tears. As a child, Sam quickly learned to suppress his feelings; it certainly was not safe. He had several experiences of being hit on the head when he was not doing what his father thought he should be doing. "But I didn't have the terrible things happen to me that others have had in their childhood," Sam told me. "I don't understand why I have had so many problems."
>
> Perhaps Sam was not abused in ways that he has read about other children. Yet, his experience, unique to him, hurt deeply. Never able to reach what he perceived as the perfection expected of him, as an adult he has been under the care of medical doctors and a psychiatrist ("basically just prescribing medication") for years. Sam suffers from anxiety, high blood pressure, irritable bowel syndrome, accelerated heart rate, chest pressure, restlessness, and stress-related outbreaks of canker sores. His stomach problems were so severe, physicians operated to remove the vagus nerve to the stomach.

Whether you begin in childhood or as an adult, if you constantly suppress yourself in order to be what someone else wants, your physical body will respond.

Emotions are real — and it takes a lot of energy to hold your Emotional Self intact. One way to do it is to stuff the feelings down with food.
It works temporarily. Eating does stuff emotions. The energy begins to rise and you can stuff it down — not express it, not feel it.

It is important to realize that if you have made decisions about being unemotional due to an overly-emotional mother or a father whose anger

179

dominated the household, you may be hurting yourself now. Analyze the difference between one whose emotions *rule* the person and one whose Emotional Self is balanced, honest, and flowing. If you had a negative role-model in this area, it may take some re-evaluation on your part. Your unconscious mind could have blockages related to expressing your Emotional Self.

Depending upon the *degree* of blockage, this could take a lot of inner work on your part. I can also tell you that it can be quite enjoyable as you begin to take steps to become aware of your feelings and to free them up. Consider how you respond to the emotions of others. Why is this important? Because it may indicate discomfort with your own emotions.

"I suppress everything," Kay said, after doing the *Body-Mind-Spirit Reflections*. "It's just easier to avoid the situation." Carol joined in, "I can be pleasant, but if I'm angry or hurt, I just grin and bear it. No one would know. It's easier to shut up. I don't like confrontation and I don't want to rock the boat." In contrast, Marie exclaimed, "You'll know exactly how I feel." Growing up in an Italian family, she was given freedom to express her emotions in a way that her friends had not experienced.

> ▲ I have a client and friend, Mona, who, over the years, has moved from being a passive, shy introvert to an independent woman with a great sense of humor who knows her own mind. During several years of inner work, she gradually stopped allowing her adult children and other family members to treat her like a doormat. And, during that process, Mona lost weight. After several years of working outside the home full time, she quit her job to stay home and begin a new career. To her shock, she began to gain more and more weight. In talking to me, she spoke of her confusion. Her relationship with her husband had improved; Mona was now valuing herself more and speaking up to him when needed. She was quite certain that she was no longer stuffing her emotions down, as she had done all of her life. Until…
>
> As a 50th birthday gift to herself, Mona decided to have braces put on her teeth to improve her bite and avoid possible problems in the future. Because of discomfort with the braces, she was unable to eat

anything but liquids for several weeks. During this time, she was *not able* to put food into her mouth. And, to her shock, the uncontrollable emotional energy that she suppressed over the years, began to rise. This was because she could no longer stuff down the anger, frustration, hurt, and disappointment with food. "Before this experience, I had no idea I was stuffing my emotions down, Janet," she said later. "I thought I was taking care of my needs and expressing my feelings very well. I found out differently. When I couldn't eat, the honesty had to come out." She is losing weight now and has additional insight into her own former *need* for excess fat.

I use this as an example because sometimes the close down of emotions can be more subtle than one might think. Feeling nervous? Eat a cookie. Frustration with your mate over dinner? Eat more than you ordinarily would. Angry over a work situation? Walk through your door and go straight to the refrigerator. To get in touch with this area, it requires paying a lot of attention to your feelings and noticing your actions over time. Sometimes a tremendous inner turmoil builds over the years. This energy force is very powerful.

More than a few women have tearfully said to me: "Why can't he love me the way I am?" After the wedding, many wives gain weight and are unable to lose it. The weight may have been a result of many factors. The *need to keep* it, however, has a connection to frustration within the marriage.

Why a *need* to keep excess fat? Because the emotions of anger and frustration and fear have been stuffed down. In order to release the emotions, she might need to force some frightening choices in the relationship. Examples could include: the risk of losing the relationship completely, losing financial security, the risk of losing friends, and feeling deserted and alone. Recognize what a very real threat this can be to a person who unconsciously believes she will forfeit her security by speaking out.

You see, your Emotional Self can feel daunted in the face of threat. Depending upon your sense of self worth, you may either be able to act in your own behalf, or chose to forfeit your power.

> **Many people are so busy being who their husbands, wives, children, parents and friends want them to be, there is no energy left to discover who they are — their likes, dislikes, and personality. As long as you are living your life for other people, your energy will be scattered. You will be drained.**

Don't misunderstand. I'm not saying that you have to leave your husband or wife in order to lose weight. Not at all. But you *may have to become more of who you are* in order to be happy, in order to stop overeating. In becoming more w*hole*, there may be changes in the way you relate to those closest to you. Are you willing to accept that they might not approve of the changes?

I have had several clients whose mothers continue to be the dominant force in their lives. I'm talking about adult women and men in their 40s or 50s who are still responding to their mother's wishes, instead of their own desires. The mother makes decisions that impact her son or daughter's entire family. An example is going to mother's for the holiday meal, even though it might be enjoyable to stay at home or start a new tradition. The conflict can be enormous. Often it *seems* easier to give in, to avoid a disturbance, and to keep peace. Do you eat *more* at family gatherings? Are you stuffing your feelings down?

When something in daily life triggers an emotion, you may be surprised at your over reaction. The over reaction is a result of the trigger *plus* the emotion which has been stored. After years of storing emotion, there can be an unrealistic fear that if you were to let it go, it would be more than an over reaction; it could possibly overtake you. If this is a concern, seek out professional support with a qualified regression therapist. I promise that the rewards will be well worth the effort.

I encourage you to get in touch with your greater self, and to enjoy the excitement of discovering your true emotional being. Don't let the pain of the past, or unconscious programming and decisions based upon poor role models, hold you back.

If you are a person with potential for a passionate, emotional zest for life, stop putting yourself into neutral. Don't stuff your own personality down to fit into what you perceive others want you to be. Someone else's approval is not worth what you are doing to your body!

Feelings and emotions add color to life. You cannot truly feel the joy of life until you allow the free-flowing energy of your Emotional Self.

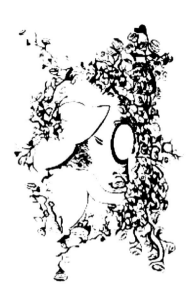

Body-Mind-Spirit Reflections- Phase 2

Δ

Your Mind and Emotions

Reflection 3 ~ Exploring Your Relationship Your SELF

Remember to write with your non-dominant hand.
How do you treat yourself? As something of value, or like a pair of old sneakers?

_____

_____

_____

_____

_____

How you treat yourself is an indication of your internal self-value. Consider your actions with food — eating healthy, nourishing food in quantities that make your body feel good, or eating junk food and stuffing yourself into discomfort?

_____

_____

_____

_____

_____

Examine your actions related to exercise. If not enough time, what or who are you giving your time to?

_____

_____

_____

_____

_____

_____

Examine how you treat yourself with rest and time for recuperating your energies. Do you make time for you?

_____

_____

_____

_____

Do you speak up for your own needs or suppress them for others?

_____

_____

_____

_____

_____

Reflection 4 ~ Exploring Your Emotional Self

Remember to write with your non-dominant hand.
First, write down any thoughts or feelings that come into your mind as you think about your own emotional nature.

_____

_____

_____

_____

_____

Now, let someone who you consider highly emotional come into mind. Do you have negative or positive feelings as you think about this person? Write them down.

_____

_____

_____

_____

Now, let's go to your childhood or teen years. What messages, verbal and nonverbal, did you receive about your emotions? Specifically, let's look at your —

Anger:

_____

_____

_____

_____

Fear:

_____

_____

_____

_____

_____

Messages about sadness:

_____

_____

_____

_____
_____

How did you act out your frustration and what messages did you get about your actions?

_____
_____
_____
_____
_____

To what degree were you able to express excitement and enthusiasm?

_____
_____
_____
_____
_____

What messages did you receive about your emotions related to love? For example, as a child, who gave or wanted hugs, and love and attention — the expression of such feelings?

_____
_____
_____
_____
_____

What messages did you receive about your sexuality? Consider your *emotional* reaction.

_____

_____

_____

_____

_____

Reflection 5 ~ Decisions Related to Your Emotional Self

Continue writing with your non-dominant hand.

Think about your husband or wife, child or parent. Allow yourself to think of a time in which this person was very sad, or angry, or boisterous and loud. After you have given yourself time to think about various situations, write down your feelings:

_____

_____

_____

_____

_____

Think of another instance when you might have been on the receiving end of another person's emotions. Write down your feelings *and* your actions. What did you do?

_____

_____

_____

_____

Look at what you have written. What are you learning about your Emotional Self?

_____

_____

_____

_____

Your Spiritual Self

Δ

The Connection to Mind

What is your Spiritual Self? The source of our spirit is the God-Energy, in whatever way a person views God. Your Spiritual Self is the link between God and your physical self. Similar to the energy of your emotions and the energy of your mind, the energy of your spirit is not visible.

Consider this: there are some people who you love to be around; they just make you feel good. Such people could be full of vitality and sparkle, or might be calm, quiet, and soothing. Whatever their personality, the energy that you sense is positive and loving. And you might be aware of people who you prefer to avoid or get away from as fast as possible. Their energy is not compatible with yours; you might sense it as angry, hateful, or negative. Those personalities are being reflected by that person's spirit. The spirit may not be physically seen, however, its presence can be strongly felt.

As we discussed earlier, the way a person *thinks* is reflected in the physical body. A person who is overburdened and feels the heaviness of life bearing down, walks and holds his or her body in a different manner from one who is in the midst of an exciting and fun-filled new life venture. In like manner, one's *emotions* are reflected in the physical body. The person experiencing sorrow and grief looks quite different from the person experiencing anger, jealousy or love.

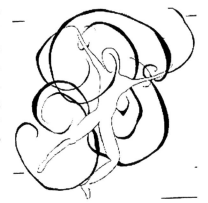

Your Spiritual Self is your higher essence — your highest being. It is affected by your childhood experiences, your environment, and the energy of others.

> **You can hide behind the words you speak.**
> **You can mask your feelings by covering an honest reaction.**
> **You cannot, however, fake your spirit.**

If our spirit is burdened with long-term storage of negativity, it cannot shine forth as its true bright light.

As mentioned, overweight people tend to be highly intuitive and sensitive. In fact, you are much more sensitive to other people's energy at an *unconscious* level than you might realize. I have discovered that a majority of overweight clients are highly sensitive, not only to themselves, but also to the energy of others.

Have you ever walked into a room where there was one person with his or her back to you and you immediately sensed sadness or anger? You had not seen their face; no words had been spoken. How did you feel or know? If you have had this or a similar experience, it is your own sensitive nature picking up on another person's energy.

> **When you connect to your Spiritual Self, you connect to your sensitivity.**
> **Your *spiritual energy* is attuned to much more than**
> **your intellect acknowledges.**

It's not spooky, or foreign, or dangerous. It is a reality of vibrational energy. What makes you stand a certain distance from an open fire? You sense the energy, the heat.

> **Call it instinct, gut reaction, intuition, or sixth sense.**
> **The ability to sense beyond the physical is innate in all of us.**

If you are a mother, you might recognize this instinct through the connection that you had when your children were babies and could not speak; you were able to intuit their needs. If you are a business executive, you might recognize it through good judgment based on gut reaction. You might have had an experience of listening to your intuition and avoiding an accident — or *not* listening to your instincts and hiring an employee who later had to be fired.

What does all of this have to do with excess weight? If you are an intuitive-sensitive, and you are uncomfortable or do not understand this sensitivity, you will have an unconscious need to *shut it down*.

You might, in fact, be so sensitive that you are aware and can *feel* the emotions of another person. Such sensitivity will often mean that you will feel a need for protection from the onslaught of others' energy.

Let's consider this sensitivity to other people's energy. Many of my clients have recognized that they can sometimes sense what another is feeling. For example, over a cup of coffee, a distraught friend might pour out her heart to you about difficulties in a love relationship or serious problems with her children. She walks away feeling better, but you have *absorbed* her problems.

Many people are like *sponges* in their ability to pick up such negative energy from

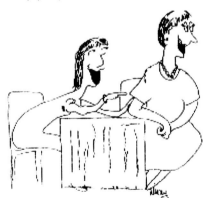 friends and family members. One particularly vulnerable client realized that after a large family or work-associated gathering, she sometimes had to go to bed to recuperate.

If this happens to you, rather than absorbing another's issues and problems, it is helpful to listen with empathy, yet in your own mind detach as in watching a movie.

Everyone has some degree of sensitivity or intuitiveness. Yet, we have not been taught to listen to it, how to value it, or put it to use. Many people are uncomfortable with their sensitive nature. Rather than viewing it as a plus, they are inclined to ignore it. In order to compensate for what they see as a flaw in their character, they move away from their sensitive nature and turn attention to their intellect. Most are able to recognize that when they do listen to their intuition, it usually pays off.

Dieters are often unable to prioritize the needs of their spirit and place an over-emphasis on the body. Their spirit is crying out for recognition, from others and themselves.

Because of the high sensitivity of many overweight people, it is my belief that diets and exercise that emphasize the body without attention to the mind and spirit will not meet their needs.

Your intuitive Spiritual Self connects to your Emotional Self which fuels feelings. It is body feelings that people desire to shut down because they can cause great pain.

> ▲ Beth remembered being taken to a hospital when she was a little girl. All that she was told by her parents and the nurses was, "Now, this won't hurt." When she came out of recovery after the operation, she hurt! She hurt a lot! Beth began to cry and the adults around her said, "You're okay." In reliving this experience in hypnosis approximately 30 years later, tears rolled down her cheeks as Beth raised her voice and yelled, "I'm not okay. They cut me!"

How do you begin to trust your own instincts and feelings if they were denied in your childhood? Most of us learned in childhood to accept the opinions of others. We were taught that other people knew what was best for us. With such training, how can you learn to trust yourself? How can you respect your own inner voice? How can you hear your own body messages? Is it any wonder that we seek answers from *the experts* for the right diet, the right exercise, the right relationship or the right career?

Most of us never had the opportunity to know or listen to our inner selves. We continue to respond to the outward influence of the people around us. In so doing, we avoid the wisdom of our own inner guidance. . The way to assure that you can hear your intuition is to allow your sensitivity to be heightened.

Your Spiritual Self is a direct link to your intuition, which connects to your vibrational energy, and also to others. If you have a tendency to dull that sixth sense, drugging yourself with food will accomplish it. That is because fat serves as a protective layer which lowers the sensitivity level.

> ▲ Beth, mentioned above, was 100 lbs. overweight and recognized that her spirit was starving. "I feel like I'm made up of everything everyone wanted me to be. I'm afraid if I lose weight, I'll lose myself. I'm not important." When Beth first came to me, she was excited about opening to a new awareness of her spiritual being. She sought out books and tapes, workshops and people who were seeking their spiritual path. A couple of years later, when she looked back on that time period, she said, "I became a 'seminar junkie,' running around to all those activities. I was really running away. I was blaming my family for my problems." It has taken Beth several years to be able to be alone in her own home — to be comfortable with herself.

Another factor related to the Spiritual Self is a desire to keep one's inner being hidden safely away, where it won't be hurt. You avoid your own *integration* of body-mind-spirit by refusing to let your true Spiritual Self be revealed. Letting your true spiritual nature out is a risk that cannot be taken easily, especially if you are fearful. In order to avoid that risk, first you need to strengthen your sense of self and more highly value who you are. Then, you can draw upon your spiritual energy more fully and express it through your personality.

**When you understand the *reasons* why you have a
need for fat at an unconscious level, you can
re-evaluate whether you still want to keep it.**

The God-Force is the Source of all and is an expression of love. Therefore, your own Spiritual Self is love and seeks love. If, however, your personality feels as if something is missing or you wonder, "Is this all there is?", you may be sensing your own spiritual quest. Love? You are wondering about weight and I'm talking about love? Yes, of course love of yourself is what I'm discussing. Love is your link to the Source.

As you move through your blockages in mind and spirit, you will become clearer. Your energy will be more free-flowing and expressive. You will no longer stop yourself by putting up barriers. You will become who you are meant to be.

When you clear away the negative energy, you heighten the awareness of intuitive wisdom. Your body needs are sensed through that knowing. These impulses of intuition are the guidance for your body's needs and can only come in the present moment.

Your body's needs throughout the day will shift and change according to your circumstances, both externally and internally. Learn to listen in the *present moment*. Those best-laid plans for healthy eating often disappear under stressful situations. For example, if you are not attuned to your body, tension at work due to a project could lead you to the snack machine and skipping lunch. A young mother who feels overwhelmed might ignore the healthy salad she planned, and instead eat the leftovers from her children's plates and the pan on the stove.

In these examples, taking a brief break at work, or taking your children outside to clear your tension, could be a solution to help you come back to a centered space. You cannot know in advance what your entire day involves and your emotional response to the situations in your life. Learn to stay attuned to your body, and listen to the intuitive guidance that it gives. A good question to ask is, *What does my body need right now for health and peace?*

Your Spiritual Self is more Light, more Love.
When you feel more *Light*, you become more *Light*.
Your body feels lighter and you want to eat lighter.

I encourage you to let your true Light shine...You are loved!

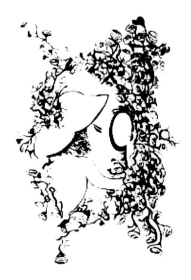

Body-Mind-Spirit Reflections-
Phase 3

Δ

Your Spiritual Self

Reflection 6 ~ Exploring Your Spiritual Self

Remember to write with your non-dominant hand.

How do you feel about your intuition?

_____
_____
_____
_____
_____
_____

How are you using your intuition?

_____
_____
_____
_____
_____

How do you listen to your Inner Self for guidance?

_____

_____

_____

_____

_____

What ways do you avoid listening to your inner guidance?

_____

_____

_____

_____

_____

Do you trust your instincts...or do you want for someone else to tell you what is right for you?

_____

_____

_____

_____

_____

Do you make time daily for prayer or meditation, walking in nature, or in some way connecting to something greater than yourself? If not, what are ways that you can begin to do this?

_____

_____

_____

_____

Reflection 7 ~ Listening to Your Inner Spirit

Remember to write with your non-dominant hand.

Be receptive to your intuitive side. What does your *intuition* (not what your conscious mind thinks you "should" do) tell you about your personal next step in your weight management program?

_____

_____

_____

_____

_____

Mentally:

_____

_____

_____

_____

_____

Emotionally:

_____

_____

_____

_____

_____

Spiritually:

_____

_____

_____

_____

_____

Reflection 8 ~ Taking Action in My World
Remember to write with your non-dominant hand.

I sense that my body now needs:

_____
_____
_____
_____
_____

Therefore, I am going to:

_____
_____
_____
_____
_____

Something that would *feel good* to my physical body would be:

_____
_____
_____
_____
_____

Therefore, I am:

_____
_____
_____
_____

Something that would *feel good* to nourish my Mental Self would be:

_____
_____
_____

_____

_____

_____

Therefore, I am:

_____

_____

_____

_____

Something that would *feel good* to my Emotional Self would be:

_____

_____

_____

_____

Therefore, I am:

_____

_____

_____

_____

A way for me to nourish my Spiritual Self would be:

_____

_____

_____

_____

Therefore, I am:

_____

_____

_____

_____

Your Spirit - We Speak!

Δ

Your Body as a Sacred Vessel

We believe that your body is a *sacred vessel* which houses your soul[2] during your existence here on earth. The conscious care and tending you give your body (i.e., physical energy form) can facilitate your soul's work while on earth. This attention can lift you to a higher level of spiritual development and accelerate your soul's journey.

> **Developing an awareness of your biochemical health can expand your spiritual energy form.**

What you feed your body also feeds your spirit. Becoming more aware of this connection can be motivating. Your biochemistry is the *nutritive river* which feeds every cell of your body. The quality of nutrient compounds that is provided to your cells, from diet, determines the quality of new body tissue that is created, for better or for worse. The biochemical impact on your cells — whether it is nutritive-based or thought-based — determines good health or lack of health. Consistent care of your body as well as your mind not only improves your physical energy form, it can free your spirit to evolve to its full potential.

> **The very act of honoring and feeling gratitude for our sacred vessel imprints positively at the biochemical level.**

It can be inspiring to recognize that your body (enveloping sheath) is a temporary home for your soul. Your soul is intricately woven into all of your energy forms in a way that may be perceived as a hologram. Your soul speaks to you through the

---

[2] For our purposes in this chapter, we may use the words "soul" and "spirit" interchangeably.

wisdom of your body. Are you listening? Your body speaks to you revealing its wisdom. We encourage you to maintain good health and look to your body for intuition and spiritual insight.

When the health of your body and mind are diminished, your spirit is affected. Being distracted by a sick body may deter the soul's work. Negativity can arise out of continually *feeling bad.* Well-known psychologist Abraham Maslow's theory of self-actualization indicates that we cannot *self actualize* until our fundamental support systems are secure. This would include food, shelter, safety, and we would add, *good physical health.*

Alternatively, your spirit can soar when your body is in harmony. Vibrant physical and mental energy forms offer a sacred space for spiritual development. When you are able to merge body, mind and spirit, you can teach your intellect to listen to and serve your body. In so doing, your personality can become consciously connected to your spirit.

> **Through lifestyle choices, such as nutrition and diet, exercise patterns, stress management, spiritual reflection and meditation, you can become a more aware participant in your soul's journey!**

Your Mind is a Sacred Bridge Linking Body and Spirit

Your mind encompasses all of your energy forms. The mind is an important link between body and spirit. Just as with the body — what you feed it determines its health — so it is also true how you feed the mind determines *its* health.

What do you feed your mind? Do you feed it with negative self-talk? Do you focus it on the weaknesses and disappointments from others? Does your mind dwell in fear, anger, judgments, or scarcity? In what kind of an environment does your mind exist? Who do you spend time with? One's chosen surroundings can encourage growth or prompt deterioration.

When you obsess over disappointments, you are often pulled into fear or anger. These are lower vibrations. If your mind is pulled down into negativity, you cannot, at the same time, be aware of your connection to spirit. On the other hand, if your mind is being uplifted with higher thoughts, joyful company, music, fun, and other positive input, it is easier to become aware of the higher vibrations emanating from your spirit.

What you spend time with determines whether or not you are building your sacred bridge between your physical body and your spirit. This bridge was actually started before your birth. The joining of the spirit to the physical takes place at some point when the spirit comes in and joins with the fetus. Even at this point, your mind, or consciousness, is aware.

Research tells us that in the womb the developing fetus has consciousness. In fact during that development, we have two streams of consciousness. One is that of a less aware, developing fetus. The other is that of a higher and more mature awareness, often referred to as the *higher self* or your *spirit*. A completely new being is created that combines the genealogy of your ancestry with the totality of your spirit. This was the beginning of your life — the joining of your spirit in the physical world.

Repairing the Ancestral Bridge

In order to get a sense of how vast the mind-bridge is, it may help to understand some points about your ancestral genealogy. Before birth, your fetus was developing with all of the genes from your mother and father, from your mother's mother and her father, from your father's mother and his father, from your grandmother's mother and her father's parents, from your father's.....well, you get the picture.

Are you familiar with the trials and challenges of your ancestors? Well, like it or not, those ancestral memories are a part of the *holographic you*. The gene pool goes back...further and further back.

An increasing number of mental health experts are finding that encoded in our DNA are the characteristics of our ancestors. In addition to your personal experiences growing up, you also carry within you the complete timeline of your ancestral characteristics. These can include cultural patterns and beliefs, and even the mental and emotional experiences of your ancestors. We point out the ancestral connection because we believe that when we are aware, it helps us to grasp more of who we are. Self awareness can be a powerful tool in strengthening the bridge that links us to our higher self.

In many ancient cultures, there was a harmonious balance between nature and Spirit, between the earth and its Creator. In modern times, that mind-bridge has become strained as we have lost our connection to our ancestors and to the land. In today's world, for many people, harmony and connection to nature and spirit has disappeared. You may unconsciously long for that harmony which brings wholeness and inner peace. In some cases, you may seek to fill that emptiness with extreme behavior that can result in self-abuse or addictions.

Each of us has the ability to tap into our higher-spirit knowing through conscious, ongoing positive attention to our thoughts, our emotions, and our body. This requires simplifying our lives and taking time for balancing techniques such as personal reflection, prayer, meditation, and silent time alone. These techniques actually calm the nervous system, relax the mind, allow the stress (adrenal) glands to rest, and shift the biochemistry in a positive manner. They also connect us to the unconscious and intuitive perspective, expanding our awareness and vision.

Daily time for these important balancing tools help us to repair the connection between body and spirit. We are calling this connection the *mind-bridge*. When the mind-bridge is strong, there is a wholeness felt within the entirety of our being. We can then perceive, with more clarity, the guidance of our spirit. This is especially so during life changes.

Healthy Cycles of Change

Changes of life are a natural progression of maturing and can be honored with excitement and joy. What we believe about the aging process and how we perceive it will manifest either a positive or negative continued life experience. This is true for both men and women.

Many men experience a *mid-life crisis*. They may struggle with heightened emotional sensitivity, begin to resist the unrelenting stress of wage earner and long for freedom from job and family pressures. Allowing the embracement toward a more feeling-emotional life can free the maturing man to create a lifestyle brimming with newfound pleasures.

Of course the change of life for a woman is more easily recognized. Due to menses, a woman is more in tune with her body and the cycles of nature. Later in life, the shift from child-bearing years creates distinct physical and biochemical changes. In the past, these changes were accepted as a natural process. However, in our society, change of life for women is tainted with negative connotations.

Sadly, menopause today is viewed as a medical condition complete with physical and emotional symptoms. Has this confusion over natural cycles occurred because we have lost our connection to nature and spirit?

This societal paradigm is not universal. In fact, in cultures where life flows with nature and spirit, the mature years are honored. Aging is revered and is celebrated as the culmination of wisdom gained throughout life.

Whenever the body's natural changes are not acknowledged, imbalances occur and symptoms appear. These are warnings to call us back into balance. The menopausal symptoms that we consider common in our society are not at all common in traditional cultures. Researcher Margaret Lock discovered that there is no single word which represents *hot flash* in the Japanese language. This is also true for the Navaho language. Have you noticed that most of the words in the English language around menopause and aging appear to be negative?

Is it possible that our symptoms today may result from a lack of respect for our natural cycles? In a comparative study of Greek and Mayan women, no Mayan woman reported hot flashes or sweats. Symptoms such as anxiety, negative attitude, and female health concerns were associated with child-bearing years, but not with menopause. Mayan women welcomed menopause with expressions such as: *free like a young girl again, happy with good health.* Greek women, on the other hand, reported symptoms such as those common to industrialized societies, including the United States. This included hot flashes, night sweats, depression, anxiety, and weight gain.

It was found that women in veiled societies actually look forward to becoming menopausal. Because they are past the child-bearing years, they can come out from behind the veil and take a more active role in community affairs. In many societies, women actually gain in status with advanced age. The cessation of menses is a milestone in that regard. In those cultures, older women are revered and elevated as wise consults. This is radically different from western societies where her status decreases as she ceases to be fertile.

People in our society tend to dread the aging process, viewing this natural cycle as a passing of their prime. Many western women feel they no longer have much to look forward to after menopause, as they age.

> ▲ Janet remembers a client, Cathy, who at age 53, told her, "I feel like my life is over." Her children were grown. She had no career, healthy relationship or life purpose. It seemed as if Cathy's spirit was expiring. It is sad that at such a young age, she could not visualize the vast opening available to her. She was standing at the cusp of her next life cycle!

Research indicates that one's attitude towards menopause is a determinant of symptomotology. As we have seen, women in western-industrialized cultures tend to report more symptoms than women in more traditional societies. When we recognize, trust and believe that changes are part of the natural life process, we will manifest fewer symptoms and feel healthier. Our later life cycle can also be a time for welcoming new creative forces within us. The post-menopausal years can enhance a women's connection to her emotional body.

▲ One client, Julia, told Judith that she may have to stop wearing eye make-up. "I feel emotions so deeply now, that I am often watery-eyed and my mascara keeps running. I love having the emotional surges, but not the black eyes."

These emotions connect us more strongly to our intuition. Acknowledging and allowing emotions, listening to our intuition, and respecting healthy cycles of change all work to strengthen the bridge to our spirit.

Integrating Body, Mind and Spirit

When we speak of our spirit or soul, we intuitively recognize that there is an aspect of us that exists beyond the physical. Today's research in consciousness supports this concept. Research in near-death experiences and regression to early memories has gathered a wealth of evidence to support the long-held belief that consciousness resides inside and also beyond the physical body.

As you recognize the holographic nature of your being, the consciousness that goes beyond your physical body is what is often referred to as your spirit. And, as explained earlier, your spirit can be hurt, resulting in lowered self-esteem and a belief that you do not deserve happiness and success in life.

How does this fit into your weight management plan? More important than how much you weigh is the wellness of your entire Being. Everything that you take into your body, including your environment and what you place your attention on, affects your spirit.

Your spirit is within you, yet is also so much vaster. You are encompassed in your own greater spirit energy form. You walk within that spirit energy form.

When you are consciously connected to Universal Oneness,
you become more aware of the Majesty of your Being.

A Practical Checklist
to Alter your Physical Journey

With a deeper understanding, you can now give priority to manifesting greater health. The bullets listed below may help propel you in that direction.

Take stock of your physical health.
▲ Develop your own health history record.
▲ Seek intervention and support on a regular basis.

Eat consciously and provide nutrients daily to your body.
▲ Consume foods daily that are highest in nutrients (nutrient dense).
▲ Consume a raw food serving with every meal; foods with a life-force have the highest available nutrients.
▲ Choose beverages that are nourishing, not depleting, such as herbal teas, diluted fruit juices, and pure water.
▲ Supplement nutrients to compensate for the less than perfect diet.
▲ Give thought to what you put on your skin. The skin absorbs directly into the blood stream. Avoid using products containing mineral oil, waxes, SD 40 alcohol, lanolin, animal by-products, excessive preservatives and synthetic colors and fragrances.
▲ Choose skin care products that contain plant compounds and essential oils.

Cleansing the body opens intuitive channels. Consider:
▲ Detoxing through periodic cleanses using sweat baths and saunas.
▲ Supporting your system, especially the liver, by using herbal supplementation.
▲ Inner-body cleansing by upgrading the diet. As soon as you improve the quality of the diet, stored toxins begin to be released.
▲ Supporting your liver, a major toxin-eliminating organ, by omitting the following, especially during cleansing treatments:
  ▪ Certain foods and beverages, such as refined sugars and starches (white flour foods), unhealthy fats, caffeine, alcohol, chemical drinks such as sodas, and other processed drinks.

207

- Synthetic chemical compounds: pesticides, additives, synthetic hormones, and over-the-counter drugs; seek out herbal remedies.
- Be sure to work with a practitioner familiar with cleansing treatments.

Developing a body movement program helps you maintain good health.

▲ Seek the assistance of a personal trainer to help get started.
▲ Be consistent with variety and have fun. This provides an enjoyable connection to your body.

Manage stress.

▲ Take steps before pathologies develop.
▲ Schedule downtime weekly to rejuvenate.
▲ Get adequate sleep and rest. Many study outcomes recommend at least eight hours of sleep per night.

Communicate with and listen to your spirit.

▲ Learn to pay attention, trust, and follow your intuition.
▲ Experiment with music, dance and song, aromatherapy, therapeutic baths, massage, yoga and tai chi.
▲ Communicate with Spirit through prayer and personal reflection.
▲ Listen to wisdom of Spirit through meditation, nature walks, and being in silence.
▲ BE JOYFUL. HAVE FUN!

Your presence, your words, your actions, and what you do with your life, affects your soul. It affects your children and their children and their children's children. Don't waste your life — live it fully!

Appendix

A

Calorie & Gram Counter for 50 Favorite Foods

We realize that lives today are enormously busy and the fact is, most of us choose foods from among our 50 favorites. To make the *gram and calorie counting aspect of the plan simpler*, use the following form to list your 50 favorite foods with their calorie and gram levels.

Enter below (or on separate pages) your favorite foods. Look them up in *The Complete Book of Food Counts*, by Corinne Netzer, and list next to each entry the gram and calorie count for each item listed. Later, when you are in a hurry, you will have a quick resource in your workbook for entering foods and amounts in your Daily Diary.

We understand that recording your daily food and beverage intake can be a challenge. Keep in mind, however that *we are educating ourselves as to why weight-loss maintenance has not been successful in the past*. To that end, personal responsibility can only take place when knowledge is also present.

When you are working to maintain weight levels, it is important to keep a daily and weekly check on how many calories you are consuming so it doesn't *get away* from you. The example below illustrates how to record your grams and calories.

Breakfast

Food Item   Carb g Protein g Fat g   Total Calories

Lunch

Food Item   Carb g Protein g Fat g   Total Calories

Dinner

Food Item   Carb g Protein g Fat g   Total Calories

Snacks

Food Item   Carb g Protein g Fat g   Total Calories

Making the Math Easy
Finding the 40-30-30 Balance

Add the total grams (carbs/protein/fats) for your meal. Then divide each part by the *total* grams to get the percentage for that part.

Carb grams divided by Total grams = % of Carbs
Protein grams divided by Total grams = % of Protein
Fat grams divided by Total grams = % of Fat

Remember, we recommend a dietary intake of 40% from the Carbohydrate food group, 30% from the Protein food group, and 30% from the Fat food group.

Do's and Don'ts for Eating Out

Do:

- Order seafood, chicken, turkey, or lean beef
- Ask that food be prepared baked, pan-fried, grilled, or broiled
- Ask for the vegetable of the day, and add a salad
- Get a side of olive oil and lemon for your salad
- If olive oil is not available, ask for a side of mayonnaise, crumbled egg, guacamole, yogurt or sour cream to blend in
- Order a baked potato or red skinned potatoes
- Ask for sandwiches on whole-grain bread
- Choose bottled or mineral water
- Put lemon in your water — lemon is an anti-bacterial

Don't:

- Eat at fast-food restaurants
- Eat salad dressing, unless it is made from olive oil
- Order deep-fried food, including French fries or chips
- Eat pasta dishes
- Drink the water, unless it is filtered
- Add restaurant salt, which is unbalanced sodium-chloride
- Order sandwiches on white bread
- Be afraid to substitute and ask for what you want!

Gluten Containing Grains

Barley
Bulgur wheat
Cous cous
Cracked wheat
Durham or Semolina wheat
Graham flour
Kamut (relative of durham wheat)
Oats & Oatmeal
Orzo and Farina
Rye
Spelt
Tabouli
Triticale (wheat and rye hybrid)
Wheat, Wheat berries, and Whole wheat
Wheat bran, Wheat germ

Grains Without Gluten

Amaranth
Buckwheat (kasha)
Corn (hard on the intestines; avoid if you have irritable bowel syndrome [IBS])
Millet (contains no gluten, but has sugars that are difficult for Celiacs to digest)
Quinoa (pronounced keenwa)
Rice — white, brown and wild

- Avoid gluten grains if you have mucous-related disorders (e.g., sinusitis, bronchitis, pneumonia, cold viruses, allergies and so on).

- A helpful book for GI tract problems, IBS, Celiac, Colitis, Crohn's, etc. is *Breaking the Vicious Cycle* by Elaine Gottschall BA, M.Sc.

Gluten Flour Substitutes

Read labels. The content of these flours must be 100% authentic; be certain the ingredients are not a combination of different flours (e.g., artichoke flour *and* wheat flour), especially the flours you are trying to avoid. In general, those with GI tract distress should minimize all flour foods.

Amaranth flour
Artichoke flour
Buckwheat or Kasha flour
Potato flour
Quinoa flour
Rice flour
Soy flour (some people are allergic or sensitive to soy)
Tapioca flour

Guide to Nutritional Supplements

We have observed good results over the years in working with a variety of supplement lines. Those include Arbonne International, Garden of Life, Mega Foods, and Radiant Life. In addition, doctor's lines such as Allergy Research, Biotics Research, and Metagenics have also been helpful for certain needs.

During the last two years we have personally used and suggested to clients a variety of products by Arbonne International. These products, available to the general public, and botanically-based and formulated in Switzerland, are a good example of high-quality nutritionals. The entire line is formulated to ensure that you receive the benefits of maximum absorption. We have also observed excellent results from Arbonne's well researched and scientifically advanced herbal formulas, including their weight-loss herbal formula. These products have served the health needs of many of our clients.

In the case of herbal formulas, it is important to choose those that are standardized. This means that each bottle always contains the measured ingredients as labeled. If not standardized, the levels may vary greatly. Seek out manufacturers who utilize only the highest quality ingredients. Nutritional products on the market today can vary widely as to their level of quality. The buyer needs to do his or her own research in order to choose safely.

Be aware that choosing nutritional supplements off the shelf, without the assistance of a trained and knowledgeable individual, can result in no benefit or can create symptoms.

Always check with your physician before taking nutritional supplements. Certain nutrients may be in conflict with certain prescription drugs you may be taking.

Serena's Weekly Weigh-In Report

'Example of actual client weekly weigh-in results

Week	Date	Loss/Gain	Total Loss	Weight	Measurements:				
					Bust	Waist	Stomach	Hips	Thigh
1				230					
2	2/29/04	-5	-5	225					
3	3/7/04	-4	-9	221					
4	3/14/04	-5	-14	216					
5	3/21/04	0	-14	216					
6	3/28/04	+4 /Water	-10	220	48	41.5	50	49	30.6
7	4/4/04	-2 /Cycle	-12	218					
	4/6/04	-2	-14	216					
8	4/11/04	-1	-15	215	47.5	41	49	48.5	30.1
9	4/18/04	0	-15	215					
10	4/25/04	+4 /Water	-11	219					
11	5/2/04	-2	-13	217	47	40	48	48	28.8
12	5/7/04	-2 /Cycle	-15	215					
	5/9/04	-3	-18	212	47	39.5	47.5	48	28.8
13	5/16/04								
14	5/23/04								
15	5/30/04								
16	6/6/04								
Total			18.0						

215

Resources

Food & Nutrition Products Manufacturer Information:

Advanced Health Solutions
800-943-0054
Colon health books; Acidophilus; ProFlora

Anabol Naturals
305-757-7733
Amino Balance; crystalline free-form amino acids

Arbonne International
410-897-9339
http://www.doctorsapproach.myarbonne.com
Safe, herbal weight-loss products; pure, botanically-based cosmetics;
  comprehensive nutritionals and standardized herbals; bio-identical
  progesterone cream

Biotics Research
800-437-1298
http://www.bioticsresearch.com
Amino Acid Quick Sorb – liquid free form amino acids; essential fatty acids;
  emulsified oil-soluble vitamins

CWR Environmental Products, Inc.
800-444-3563
http://www.cwenviro.com
Ceramic water-filtration systems

Eden Foods, Inc.
888-424-3336
http://www.edenfoods.com
High quality green teas

The Grain and Salt Society
1-800-TOP-SALT
http://www.celtic.seasalt.com
Unrefined sea salt offering full-spectrum, naturally balanced,
  high nutritional mineral content

Green Pastures Dairy
218-384-4513
http://www.greenpasturesdairy.com
Grass-fed cheese and meat products; nitrate and MSG-free

Honey Gardens Apiaries, Inc.
800-416-2083
http://www.honeygardens.com
Raw honey

Mega Food
800-848-2542
http://www.megafood.com
Food-formed nutritionals

Metagenics, Inc.
100 Avenida La Pata
San Clemente, CA 92673
800-692-9400
http://www.metagenics.com
Herbs and supplements available only through medical practitioners

Organic Valley Butter
608-625-2602
http://www.organicvalley.com
European-style cultured butter

Radiant Life
888-593-8333
http://www.4radiantlife.com
Norwegian cod liver oil, coconut oil; baby formula ingredients; Celtic salt

White Egret Farms
512-276-7408
http://www.whiteegretfarm.com
Grass-fed goat yogurt and cheeses; organically-raised beef and turkey

Health Organizations & Publications:

The Academy of Natural Therapies
http://www.PowerHealth.net
Study nutrition therapies in-home

American Anorexia Bulimia Association (AABA)
165 West 46th Street, Ste. 1108
New York, NY 10036
212-575-6200
http://www.aabainc.org

American Association of Nutritional Consultants
302 East Winona Avenue
Warsaw, IN 46580
888-828-2262
http://www.aanc.net
Offers certified nutritional counseling (CNC) certification

American Preventative Medical Association
9912 Georgetown Pike, Ste. D-2
Great Falls, Virginia 22066
800-230-2762
http://www.apma.net

Bastyr University
14500 Juanita Drive, NE
Kenmore, WA 98028
425-823-1300
http://www.bastyr.edu
Cancer Treatment Centers of America

Clayton College of Natural Health
2140 11th Avenue, South, Ste. 305
Birmingham, AL 35205
800-995-4590
Degree programs in nutrition

Designs for Health Institute
1750 30th Street, Ste. 319
Boulder, CO 80301
303-415-0229
http://www.dfhi.com
Training in clinical nutrition

Feingold Association of the United States
127 East Main Street, Ste. 106
Riverhead, NY 11901
800-321-3287
http://www.feingold.org
Diets for children with attention deficit disorders

Health Wisdom for Women
Dr. Christiane Northrup
207-846-3626
http://www.drnorthrup.com
Monthly newsletter discussing women's health issues

The John R. Lee, M.D. Medical Letter
800-528-0559
www.johnleemd.com
Monthly alternative health newsletter, particularly natural hormone
  therapies and progesterone research

Susan Love, M.D.
http://www.SusanLovemd.com
Excellent reference site on breast cancer

Midwestern Regional Medical Center
2501 Emmaus Avenue
Zion, IL 60099
800-615-3055
http://www.cancercenter.com
Nutrition-oriented cancer treatment

Water Quality Association
4151 Naperville Road
Lisle, IL 60532
708-505-0160
http://www.wqa.org
Information on types of water and methods of treatment

The Weston A. Price Foundation
4200 Wisconsin Avenue, NW
Washington, DC 20016
202-333-HEAL
http://www.WestonAPrice.org
Nutrition information and articles on fats, nutrient-dense foods,
  sustainable farming, research on soy
Wise Traditions in Food, Farming and the Healing Arts
Quarterly newsletter
e-mail: WestonAPrice@msn.com

Bibliography & Recommended Reading

Airola, Paavo. *Every Woman's Book*. Phoenix: Health Plus Publishers, 1979.

Bajulaiye, O. and Sarrel, P.M. "A Survey of Premenopausal Women in Nigeria," and Samil, R.S. "The Menopause in Various Cultures." *1984 International Congress on the Menopause. The Climacteric in Perspective*. MTP Press Ltd., 1986.

Balch, James, F. and Phyllis A. *Prescription for Nutritional Healing*. Avery Publishing Company, 2000.

Baussan, Olivier and Chibois, Jacques. *Olive Oil: A Gourmet Guide*. Paris: Flammarion, 2000.

Beyenne, Yewoubdar. *From Menarch to Menopause: Reproductive Lives of Peasant Women in Two Countries*. State University of New York, 1989.

Bieler, Henry, M.D. *Food Is Your Best Medicine*. Ballantine Books, 1966.

Bland, Jeffrey, Ph.D. "The Use of Complementary Medicine for Healthy Aging." *Alternative Therapies*, Volume 4, No. 4, July 1988.

Bland, Jeffrey, Ph.D. "Improving Intercellular Communication in Managing Chronic Illness." *HealthComm International, Inc.*, Seminar Series Syllabus, 1999.

Brand-Miller, Jennie, et al. *The Glucose Revolution*. Marlowe & Company, 1999.

Colgan, Michael. *Your Personal Vitamin Profile*. New York: Quill, 1982.

Cunningham, Janet. *Inner Selves: The Feminine* Path to Weight Loss (*for men and women who value their intuitive nature)*. Montreal: The Chestnut Press, 1993.

Cunningham, Janet. "The Feminine Yin Approach to Weight Loss." *Imprint Magazine*. Alberta, Canada, Issue 4, 2002.

duToit, B.M. "Cross Cultural Perspectives." *1984 International Congress on the Menopause, The Climacteric in Perspective.* MTP Press Ltd., 1986.

Enig, Mary G. "Exclusive Interview: Discussing Partially Hydrogenated Vegetable Oils." *Nutrition & Healing,* February 1995.

Enig, Mary G. Ph.D. and Sally Fallon. "Diet and Heart Disease: Not What You Think," and "The Oiling of America." *Nexus Magazine,* December 1998–January 1999, and February 1999–March 1999.

Enig, Mary G. Ph.D. *Know Your Fats: The Complete Primer for Understanding the Nutrition of Fats, Oils, and Cholesterol.* Bethesda Press, June 2001.

Fallon, Sally and Mary Enig, Ph.D. *Nourishing Traditions.* ProMotion Publishing, 1999.

Figtree, Dale. *Eat Smart: A Guide to Good Health for Kids.* Clinton, New Jersey: New Win, 1992.

Flint, M. "The Menopause: Reward or Punishment." *Psychosomatics.* 15:161–3, 1975.

Gaby, Alan, M.D. *Preventing and Reversing Osteoporosis.* Prima Publishing Company, 1994.

Gaby, Alan, M.D. "Research Review." *Nutrition & Healing.* November 1994.

Gittleman, Ann L., M.S. *Super Nutrition for Women.* New York: Pocket Books, 1993.

Gittleman, Ann L., M.S. *Beyond Pritikin.* Bantam Books, 1996.

Gottschall, Elaine, M.Sc. *Breaking The Vicious Cycle: Intestinal Health Through Diet.* Ontario, Canada: Kirkton Press, 1994.

Haas, Elson M.D. *The Detox Diet.* Celestial Arts, 1996.

Hoffer, Abram, M.D., Ph.D. and Walker, Morton, DPM. *Putting It All Together: The New Orthomolecular Nutrition.* Keats Publishing, Inc., 1996.

Howell, Edward Ph.D. *Enzyme Nutrition.* Avery Publishing Group, 1985.

Jensen, Bernard and Anderson, Mark. *Empty Harvest: Understanding the Link Between Our Food, Our Immunity and Our Planet.* Avery Publishing Group, 1990.

Lee, John, M.D. *What Your Doctor May Not Tell You About Menopause.* Warner Books, 1996.

Lee, John, M.D., Hanley, Jesse, M.D. and Hopkins, Virginia. *What Your Doctor May Not Tell You About Premenopause.* Warner Books, 1999.

Lieberman, Shari and Bruning, Nancy. *The Real Vitamin & Mineral Book.* Avery Publishing Group, 1990.

Lock, Margaret. *Encounters with Ageing: Mythologies of Menopause in Japan and North America.* University of California Press, 1993.

Murray, Michael, N.D. *Natural Alternatives to Over-the-Counter and Prescription Drugs.* William Morrow and Company, Inc., 1994.

Murray, Michael, N.D. *Encyclopedia of Nutritional Supplements.* Prima Publishing, 1996.

Netzer, Corinne T. *The Complete Book of Food Counts.* Dell Publishing Co., 1998.

Northrup, Christiane, M.D. *Health Wisdom.* October 1995 and November 1995.

Northrup, Christiane, M.D. *The Wisdom of Menopause.* Bantam Books, 2001.

Ojeda, Linda. *Menopause Without Medicine.* Alameda, California: Hunter House, 1992.

Parfit, Michael. "Pollution: Troubled Waters Run Deep," and "Water: The Promise and Turmoil of North America's Fresh Water." *National Geographic Society*, 184:5A, 1993.

Pauling, Linus. *How To Live Longer and Feel Better*. Avon Books, 1987.

Payers, L. and Samil R.S. "The Menopause in Various Cultures." *A Portrait of the Menopause*. Parthenon, 1991.

Perricone, Nicholas, M.D. *The Wrinkle Cure*. Warner Books, 2000.

Pfeiffer, Carl C., Ph.D., M.D. *Nutrition and Mental Illness: An Orthomolecular Approach to Balancing Body Chemistry*. Healing Arts Press, 1987.

Pizzorno, Joseph, N.D. *Total Wellness*. Prima Publishing, 1998.

Pizzorno, Joseph, N.D. and Murray, Michael, N.D. *Textbook of Natural Medicine*. Churchill: Livingstone, 1999.

Ronzio, Robert A., Ph.D., CNS. *The Encyclopedia of Nutrition & Good Health*. New York, New York: Facts on File, 1997.

Ross, Julia, M.S. *The Diet Cure*. Penguin Books, 1999.

Stitt, M.S. *Beating The Food Giants*. Natural Press, 1980.

Thibodeau, Gary A. *Structure and Function of the Body*. St. Louis, Missouri: Moseby-Year Book, Inc., 1992.

Valentine, Judith. "A Nutritional Guide For A Natural Menopause." Dissertation, original copy filed with Library of Congress, January 1996.

Valentine, Judith, Ph.D. "The Trouble with Low Fat Diets." *Annapolis Holistic Health Journal*, Spring 2000.

Valentine, Judith, Ph.D. "Soft Drinks: America's *Other* Drinking Problem." *Wise Traditions in Food, Farming, and the Healing Arts.* The Weston A. Price Foundation, Volume 2, No. Two, Summer 2001.

Winters, Ruth. *Poisons in Your Food.* New York: Crown Publishers, 1991.

Wright, J. and Gaby, A. "Natural Response." *Nutrition & Healing,* May, 1995.

Wright, Jonathan, MD. "The Right Amount of Vitamin C Can Fight Disease and Add Years to Your Life." *Nutrition & Healing,* Volume 8, No. 6, June 2001.

About the Authors

Janet Cunningham, Ph.D. and Judith Valentine, Ph.D.

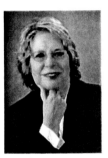

The Mind: Janet Cunningham, Ph.D. is an internationally known specialist in regression therapy, past-president of the International Association for Regression Research and Therapies, Inc., and founder and president of Heritage Authors™. Dr. Cunningham is the author of eight books including *Inner Selves: The Feminine* Path to Weight Loss* (**for men and women who value their intuitive nature*). She is owner of *Breakthroughs to the Unconscious®*, a private practice in Columbia, Maryland. Her work has been written about by other authors and featured in international magazines.

www.JanetCunningham.com

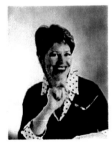

The Body: Judith Valentine, Ph.D. has worked with hundreds of clients interested in weight management and weight loss. She determines, bio-chemically, the appropriate level of supplements needed and guides clients toward safe weight-loss plans and catalysts. Dr. Valentine has lectured both on the local and national level and has written many articles featuring wellness and nutrition science. She has been on staff at Calvert Memorial Hospital's Integrative Medicine Clinic: Healthy Alternatives, and on the teaching staff at Anne Arundel Community College in Annapolis, Maryland.

www.JudithValentine.com